Saunders

Student Nurse Planner

A Guide to Success in Nursing School

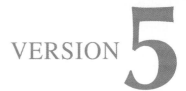

VERSION 5

Susan C. deWit, MSN, RN, CNS, PHN

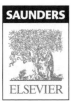

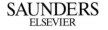

SAUNDERS
ELSEVIER

11830 Westline Industrial Drive
St. Louis, MO 63146

SAUNDERS STUDENT NURSE PLANNER, VERSION 5   ISBN: 978-1-4160-4752-0
Copyright © 2007, 2006, 2003, 1999, 1995 by Saunders, an imprint of Elsevier Inc.

Notice

Knowledge and best practice in this field are constantly changing. As new research
and experience broaden our knowledge, changes in practice, treatment and drug
therapy may become necessary or appropriate. Readers are advised to check
the most current information provided (i) on procedures featured or (ii) by the
manufacturer of each product to be administered, to verify the recommended dose
or formula, the method and duration of administration, and contraindications. It is
the responsibility of the practitioner, relying on their own experience and knowledge
of the patient, to make diagnoses, to determine dosages and the best treatment for
each individual patient, and to take all appropriate safety precautions. To the fullest
extent of the law, neither the Publisher nor the Author assumes any liability for any
injury and/or damage to persons or property arising out or related to any use of the
material contained in this book.

The Publisher

Library of Congress Control Number: 2007927259

ISBN: 978-1-4160-4752-0

Managing Editor: Robin Levin Richman
Associate Developmental Editor: Ryan Creed
Publishing Services Manager: Jeff Patterson
Senior Project Manager: Clay S. Broeker
Designer: Teresa McBryan

Working together to grow
libraries in developing countries

www.elsevier.com | www.bookaid.org | www.sabre.org

ELSEVIER   BOOK AID
International   Sabre Foundation

Printed in China
Last digit is the print number: 9 8 7 6 5 4 3 2

To the memory of
Julia Catherine Reaves
my mentor, friend, and former teaching partner,
who provided the foundation for many of the ideas
that appear in this book to help students.

Catherine's dedication to nursing, to students, and to
holistic health care for the elderly provided
continuing inspiration.

Publisher's Foreword

The student nursing experience is perhaps the most complex in the undergraduate curriculum. It entails not only the classwork and home study common to all undergraduate programs but also clinical preparations and experiences. In talking with students, nursing program administrators, and nursing classroom and clinical instructors, we found that people were looking for a general guide to help students plan and organize their time and information, particularly with respect to the clinical experience. More specifically, students and faculty were seeking the following:

▼ A portable, quick-access source of information specifically oriented to the nursing student, with brief discussions of topics such as initiating patient communication, dealing with stress, time management, emergency procedures, and basic nursing reference data

▼ A flexible 1-year planner that was not restricted to programs beginning in the fall or January only

▼ A directory for important and frequently used telephone numbers

The *Saunders Student Nurse Planner* addresses these needs.

CLINICAL INFORMATION

Chapters 1 through 6 include a general orientation to nursing school, suggestions for getting the most out of clinical rotations, tips for dealing with stress, and a broad array of useful data and procedures. Included in this edition are the following: the Glasgow Coma Scale for assessing level of consciousness, various pain assessment tools, the Body Mass Index formula for predicting obesity, a table of the characteristics of commonly used IV fluids, and information on educational opportunities for nursing careers. The information in this section was selected especially for student use in a quick reference format and has been indexed for user convenience.

CALENDARS

Both monthly and weekly calendars have been included so that students can plan out not only their short-term weekly activities but also long-term activities throughout the year. The calendars do not contain dates, so the user can write these in according to the specific beginning and end dates of the quarter or semester. Sufficient calendars have been included for one full academic year. Dated calendars in condensed form are provided for reference. Suggestions for using the calendars are included in the text portion of the planner.

TELEPHONE DIRECTORY

The telephone directory is a straightforward alphabetized directory in which to record academic and clinical instructors' names and telephone numbers and office hours, as well as information about other students to contact for missed assignments or study sessions.

We would appreciate suggestions or other feedback you may have concerning this or any of our Elsevier nursing products. Please address your comments to: Nursing Editorial, Elsevier, 1600 John F. Kennedy Boulevard, Suite 1800, Philadelphia, PA 19103-2899.

Contents

CHAPTER 3

Dealing with Stress, 65

CHAPTER 4

Continuing Your Education, 81

CHAPTER 5

Aids to Success, 85

CHAPTER 6

Obtaining Information via the Internet, 157

APPENDIX A

Nursing Outcomes Classification (NOC) Outcome Labels, 167

APPENDIX B

Nursing Interventions Classification (NIC) Intervention Labels, 171

Orientation to Nursing School

THE CHALLENGE OF NURSING SCHOOL

Nursing school is an exciting, challenging adventure that will demand much of you in terms of time and energy. Because nursing is a discipline comprising knowledge from many related fields, you will be asked to learn to think critically, synthesize information, and then apply it to situations involving live people. To learn to care correctly and safely for ill people, you must cover a large amount of information in a relatively short time. This requires efficient use of time and resources.

On Campus

Syllabus. There will be a course outline or syllabus for each nursing course (Figure 1-1). This may be available for purchase in the bookstore, handed out in class, or available on the college intranet platform to be downloaded and printed by you. When you acquire the syllabus, become familiar with the entire layout of each course. Syllabi, or course outlines, are usually divided into units of study that contain a list of learning objectives. There also may be a correlated outline of content to be covered in the unit and related learning opportunities or activities. The latter are usually readings in texts, journal articles, audiovisual presentations available at the school, computer CD or online instruction modules, and suggestions for review of material covered in earlier prerequisite classes such as anatomy and physiology.

The syllabus, or other materials handed out at the first class meeting, will state policies regarding attendance requirements, student behavior in class and clinical areas, grading criteria, dress code for clinical areas, grievance procedures, and other topics particular to each school. There will be a list of required texts and a statement about evaluation of performance for the course.

School Philosophy and Student Responsibility. Each school and nursing program has a statement of philosophy that explains how the school and instructors view the student, teaching, and learning. Most schools view the student as an active learner and the teacher as a facilitator of learning. This means that you must take responsibility for your own learning and not depend on instructors to provide all the knowledge that you need to pass a particular course.

Desired Behavior—The Student Will:	Content	Teacher/Student Activity	Selected Lab/Clinical Experience	Assignment
	UNIT V Assessment and Documentation Ch. 2 (12) Assessment and Physical Examination			
Define the vocabulary	A. Introduction	Teacher: Lecture/Discussion Student: Note Taking/Discussion		deWit, pp. 293-295
Describe the procedure for gathering data on a patient in a health care setting	B. History and Psychosocial Assessment	Video: Physical Assessment	Perform an assessment at the beginning of the shift on each assigned patient.	deWit, pp. 295-296
Describe the sequence of steps when performing physical assessment	C. Physiological Assessment 1. Methods of Gathering Information a) Observation b) Palpation c) Percussion d) Auscultation		Describe normal assessment findings. Interview a patient.	deWit, pp. 296-301
Describe information obtained in a review of basic needs	2. Nursing Assessment of Physical Functioning a) Rest/activity b) Nutrition/fluids c) Safety/security d) Hygiene e) Oxygen f) Psychosocial learning g) Elimination	Skill 12-2, p. 309 Nursing Assessment of Heart Sounds and Lung Sounds	Evaluate the interview of a selected patient.	
Describe the steps in performing a neuro check	3. Special Nursing Assessments a) Level of consciousness b) Pupillary changes c) Motor/sensory responses d) Changes in vital signs	Skill 12-3, p. 311 Neurological Check	Assist the physician with a physical examination on an assigned patient.	
Describe the sequence of events in a head-to-toe examination on a patient in a health care setting	4. Medical Physical Examination a) Positioning a patient b) Draping a patient	Skill 12-1, p. 307 Assisting with a Medical Examination	Position a patient during a physical examination.	
Explain the procedure for testing visual acuity of patients in a health care setting	D. Testing Visual Acuity	Skill 12-4, p. 313 Test for Visual Acuity		deWit, pp. 301-302

FIGURE 1-1 Example of a page from a nursing course syllabus. (From *Nursing I Syllabus 2002*, Meadville, PA, Crawford County Area Vocational-Technical School Practical Nursing Program. Reprinted with permission.)

For this reason, it is very important that you go to class prepared for the topics to be covered that day. **The prepared student has read the text pages relative to the content to be covered, taken study notes, considered the objectives to be covered, and noted questions that should be asked in class.**

During orientation to the class, the calendar of when course material will be covered by date is given to the students. Test dates and assignment due dates are set. All of this information should be entered in the *Student Planner* calendar section. This assists in organizing time and study activity.

Campus Resources. The wise student quickly becomes acquainted with the resources on campus that can make life easier. All nursing students will have access to the learning resource center, or library. Other resource areas that your campus might have include a learning or tutoring center, an adult resource center for single parents or students with special problems, students with disabilities office, counseling center, computer laboratory, audiovisual laboratory, skills laboratory, and student center. Read about these areas and services in the school catalog or student handbook. Specifically plan time to use these services and areas. Each student is entitled to the services offered in these areas through the tuition and fees paid for courses.

Some time should be scheduled each week, outside of class, for library reference work, using audiovisual material, and practicing skills. Few schools can schedule sufficient laboratory time for students to thoroughly learn a skill or enough practice time to master a skill. **Students are expected to practice more on their own time.** These activities should be scheduled in the calendar section of the *Student Planner* each week. Practice with a peer, and when the skill is mastered, have your peer critically evaluate your performance. This will help you be certain that you are ready for instructor "check-off" evaluation.

At the Hospital

The term *clinical* refers to the time the student is scheduled to be at the hospital, or other clinical site, learning to become a nurse. When you have learned the preliminary skills necessary to function in the clinical setting, you will be assigned to a clinical facility. Hospitals, long-term care facilities (nursing homes), mental health facilities, home health agencies, school health offices, and outpatient clinics are all referred to as clinical facilities. Clinical rotations may be for a day or two, a few weeks, half a semester, or a full semester. Once assigned to a clinical facility, the student may be given data about the type of patient assignment the day before the clinical experience is to take place. Otherwise specific patients are assigned at the beginning of the clinical session.

Clinical Orientation. During clinical orientation, you will be given an overview of the facility, including its size, general services, the community it serves, whether it is a public facility or a private business, the administrative structure, the physical layout, and the areas to which students will be assigned. A description of the type of nursing used on the units will be provided. Some hospitals use a team nursing approach, some use managed care, and others use primary nursing; there are many different types of care delivery. (The types of nursing will be discussed in your fundamentals of nursing course.) It is important that the student understand the division of labor among the personnel on the unit, the organization of the unit, and the lines of communication. **Also note that the patient/client is considered the "customer" and is to be treated as such.**

An orientation checklist is provided to help the student prepare to care for patients and feel more comfortable in the environment of the assigned clinical unit (Table 1-1). The list is most appropriate for a hospital unit, but can be adapted to other types of clinical facilities.

During clinical orientation, your instructor will tell you how you will receive your patient assignments for the clinical days: either your instructor will assign patients to you, or you will choose your own patients. In either event, you will need to gather data to prepare for your patient assignment. Table 1-2 provides a checklist for you to use to be certain you gather the right information.

Heavily Trafficked Areas. During orientation, students should pay attention to heavily trafficked areas to avoid obstructing the work of the unit; heavily traveled pathways and chairs where nurses or physicians need to sit to chart should be avoided at peak times of the day. Consideration will

TABLE 1-1 Clinical Facility Orientation

Meet the Personnel
▼ Unit director's and/or charge nurse's name and phone number
▼ Unit secretary's name
▼ Staff nurses', case managers', and nursing assistants' names
▼ Physicians' names

Necessary Phone Numbers (Enter These Numbers in Your *Student Planner*)
▼ Unit
▼ Dietary department
▼ Pharmacy
▼ Radiology (x-ray) department
▼ Physical therapy department
▼ Respiratory therapy department
▼ Admission office
▼ Security office
▼ Central supply room/central stores
▼ Operator
▼ Number used for emergency "code" and fire

TABLE 1-1 Clinical Facility Orientation—cont'd

Learn to Use the Equipment

▼ Learn to work the intercom system
▼ Use the Addressograph machine to imprint a piece of paper
▼ Review use of the fire extinguishers, and note alarm locations
▼ Go to a patient unit and:
  ▪ Operate all of the light switches
  ▪ Turn on and off the TV and radio; adjust the volume
  ▪ Raise and lower the whole bed; raise the head, then the foot
  ▪ Raise and lower the side rails
  ▪ Open and close the curtains
  ▪ Practice working the call light system
  ▪ Adjust the shower or bath controls
▼ Note the password for the computer if allowed to use it

Study the Environment

▼ Explore the layout of the nurses' station and find extra charting forms
  for work assignments/report sheets for work organization:
  ▪ Chart rack
  ▪ Kardex or computer patient care sheets (electronic patient record [EPR]),
    Physicians' Desk Reference
  ▪ Policy and procedure manuals
  ▪ Dietary manual
  ▪ Communication board
  ▪ Out-of-the-way areas where students can sit to chart
▼ Find all supplies that you might need for patient care; explore the supply
  cart and various cupboards
▼ Find the clean linen storage area
▼ Locate the dirty linen disposal area and the utility room
▼ Find the staff restroom
▼ Locate the patient shower or tub bathrooms
▼ Find the room where report is given
▼ Determine where to leave your coat
▼ Inquire where the student-patient assignment sheet is posted

Learn the Procedures

▼ How to access the EPR and other patient data in the computer,
  if permitted
▼ How to document care (check the documentation manual)
▼ Fire or disaster procedures
▼ Initiating an emergency "code" for cardiac or respiratory arrest
▼ Handling hazardous materials
▼ Ordering supplies for patient care and how to post charges for supplies
  and equipment used
▼ Medication administration and use of medication-dispensing machine
▼ Procedure for charting as-needed (PRN) medications and one-time
  doses
▼ Narcotic checkout procedure
▼ Special charting/reporting procedures (e.g., elevated vital signs, change
  in condition)

TABLE 1-2 Clinical Assignment Information

Diagnoses
Surgery and date performed
Vital sign schedule
Daily weight required?
Diet   I&O
Activity allowed   Degree of mobility   Traction
Type of bath required
Tubes: IV   NG   Foley   Drains   Other
Pain control method   Pain score
Medications
Allergies
Risk areas   Skin   Falls
Treatments: Dressing changes   TED hose   Heat or cold   Sitz
Physical therapy   Occupational therapy   Speech therapy
                     Respiratory therapy   TCDB
Tests ordered
Equipment in use
Prostheses
Loss of hearing   Loss of vision   Wears glasses
Any paralysis or limb weakness
Communication problems   Language spoken

I&O, Intake and output; *IV,* intravenous; *NG,* nasogastric; *TCDB,* turn, cough, and deep breathe; *TED,* thromboembolic device.

be appreciated. Whenever a chart is taken away from the immediate area of the nurse's station, notify the unit secretary where it will be in case someone needs it. Charts must be replaced exactly where they were found.

There is a push to establish "paperless" hospitals. This means that within the next decade, medical records will all be available by computer rather than sitting in a chart cover in paper form on the nursing unit. Students must become adept at accessing information about their patients on the computer.

If the facility is large and the layout is confusing, note particular landmarks on the way to the assigned unit. Try to travel to and from the unit on the same elevators each time, and note hallway decor and signs with unit and room number designations.

Some instructors assign each student to a staff nurse the first day of clinical so that they can become more comfortable and learn the usual routine of the unit. If this is not the case, becoming familiar with the new environment on orientation day will ease the fear of the unknown on the first day of actual patient care.

Preconference and Postconference. Many schools have a preconference period at the beginning of the clinical day to provide an opportunity for students to clarify assignments, ask questions, and glean moral support for the day. At the end of the clinical day most schools have a 30-minute to 2-hour clinical postconference time for discussion of the day's events, sharing of experiences, and instructor-guided learning to help meet the week's objectives. Students are often asked to do presentations on short topics, complete quizzes, or participate in group learning activities. Sometimes speakers are invited to present special topics to the clinical group.

Networking. You should begin networking with classmates and other nursing students as soon as school starts. This is how you find out what to expect in other courses, at particular clinical facilities, and from particular instructors. It is also a way to find study buddies and set up a study group. Joining the Student Nurses' Association (SNA) at your school is one way to begin. Your instructors can provide you with information about SNA meetings and phone numbers of sponsors and officers. Enter all phone numbers in your *Student Planner* directory.

SETTING UP FOR SUCCESS

Being successful in nursing school requires good time management, efficient study skills, and use of appropriate resources. The adult nursing student often has to juggle family responsibilities, work, and school, along with the miscellaneous tasks of daily life. The key to success is careful planning and as much simplification as possible in all areas of your life for the duration of the nursing program. Besides the hours spent in class and clinical, a rule of thumb for planning study time is 2 hours per week for each credit hour of the course to pass. This means that for a 3-credit-hour course, you will need to spend 6 hours studying per week to obtain a C average.

Organizing Your Time

Weekly Time Map. Coordinating all of the responsibilities and activities of day-to-day life with your school class and study schedule is essential to success in any nursing program. A good way to do this is to make a weekly time map in which you map out the time required for everything from cooking dinner or mowing the yard to picking up the children from school. The student living alone will want to coordinate time for friends, exercise, and favorite pastimes with the school schedule. The student living with family will want to set aside some time to spend with family members. Figure 1-2 shows one student's time map for 1 week. Figure 1-3 provides a blank form for your own time map. Use pencil because your first time estimates may not work. This way you can adjust the schedule until it is more accurate for each activity. Don't forget to include at least a bit of time with the important people in your life and some leisure time

TIME MAP
ACTIVITY

TIME	SUNDAY	MONDAY	TUESDAY	WEDNESDAY	THURSDAY	FRIDAY	SATURDAY
6							
7		Exercise	CLINICAL	CLINICAL	CLINICAL	Exercise	House work
8	Church or other	CLASS				CLASS	yard work etc.
9	Family Activity						Laundry ε
10							Ironing etc.
11	Brunch						
12	nap	Lunch				Lunch	Prepare week's meals
1	Study	CLASS				CLASS	
2							
3							
4		Errands Time with Kids	Errands Time with Kids	Errands CLINICAL Prep	Errands Time with Kids	Errands Study	Exercise
5	Time with Family	CLINICAL Prep	Time with husband/wife	Pick up house	Catch up time		Study
6	Dinner	Dinner	Dinner	Dinner	Dinner	out for dinner	Dinner
7	Time with Family	Time with husband/wife	Study	Study	Study	Free time	movie
8	Study	Study					etc.
9			Bed	Bed	Bed		
10	Bed						
11							
12							

FIGURE 1-2   Sample time map.

for yourself. Nothing but work and study may lead to burnout before the nursing program is completed. Enter all firm commitments, study times, and appointments in your *Student Planner* calendar. The younger college student can plan social activities, balancing that time with adequate study time. Schedule study time on the time map and work your social activity time around the school and study hours. That way your social time doesn't interfere with sufficient study. This helps set you up for success in your nursing program.

TIME	SUNDAY	MONDAY	TUESDAY	WEDNESDAY	THURSDAY	FRIDAY	SATURDAY
6							
7							
8							
9							
10							
11							
12							
1							
2							
3							
4							
5							
6							
7							
8							
9							
10							
11							
12							

TIME MAP
ACTIVITY

FIGURE 1-3 Blank time map form.

Sharing Housekeeping Tasks. If you are living in a family situation, in order to commit to the hours of study required for success in a nursing program, you need to delegate some tasks that were formerly yours to others in your household. Your partner, if you have one, can help with household chores, run errands, and help with some of the tasks of child-rearing. Children from age 4 can assist with small household tasks such as clearing the table, dusting, and putting belongings in their proper places. Children older than age 9 can cook one dinner per week (hot dogs, pancakes, or packaged macaroni and cheese are fine once in a while). Many household tasks can be delegated to this age-group, such as washing dishes, loading or emptying the dishwasher, mopping, vacuuming, weeding, raking leaves, or watering. Adolescents can cook a couple of meals a week, do the grocery shopping from a list, put the groceries away, do their own laundry, mow the lawn, wash the car, and help with household chores. If they are competent drivers, they can run errands and pick up and deliver smaller children to school or activities. Relatives can fill in for you at school functions when you are studying for an examination and can spend more special time with your children when you cannot.

Work Adjustments. Once your decision to begin work on a nursing curriculum has been made, check with your employer about the possibility of flexible hours to accommodate the need for extra study time before exams and for hospital clinical rotation requirements. Many employers do adjust hours for nursing students. To give yourself the best chance at success in the nursing program, try not to work more than 20 hours per week. If after the first few months of the program you find you have extra time when you could work, and you are doing well academically, then you may be able to increase the number of work hours. Work hours may need to be adjusted again later in the program as courses become more demanding. If your employer is not able to adjust your schedule, you may wish to find a job working as a technician or as a patient care assistant in the local hospital during your training period. Many hospitals offer tuition reimbursement and flexible schedules for nursing students. Some hospitals have scholarship funds available for employees as well.

Another temporary or part-time job is as a student assistant on campus. Most colleges have a part-time work program available for students. Placement as division "gofers," part-time secretaries or receptionists, lab helpers, classroom aides, library helpers, and the like are possibilities. These positions are limited and go to the quick applicants. The Student Development Office is the place to inquire about this type of employment.

A third possibility for part-time employment may be available for those who have a previous college degree or who excel in certain subjects such as math, English, or science. A tutor in the college learning or tutoring center can earn $9.00 an hour or more. The financial aid officer can provide information about grants and loans available and also may have scholarship information. The counseling center can assist you in a search for scholarship funds, as can both the school and local community librarian. Whatever your work schedule, enter your work hours in your *Student Planner* calendar each week.

Study Skills

The study of nursing requires a great deal of reading. If there is doubt about your reading efficiency, contact your counselor or academic adviser and arrange to have your reading skills evaluated. Once the evaluation is done, and any problem areas identified, methods by which your reading *efficiency* can be improved will be suggested. The few hours spent learning how to read more efficiently can save you much study time in the future. Also inquire about a college learning skills course. Many schools offer such a course and some gear sections specifically to health occupation students. Students have found such a class, which is usually only 1 credit hour, to be a great tool for success in the nursing program.

Learning Styles. It is also helpful to evaluate how you learn best. Some people are visual learners; others are auditory learners; and some learn best by doing, and hence are tactile or kinesthetic learners. Most students have a predominant learning mode but also use at least one of the other modes to advantage. The college learning center or the counseling center can direct you in ways to evaluate your own learning style. Once you are aware of which mode is best for you, it is possible to structure your studying around that mode. If you are a visual learner, studying texts, reading articles, and seeing visual presentations such as videos is the best way to spend your study time. If you are an auditory learner, taping lectures, listening to audiotapes from supplementary audiovisual materials, and perhaps reading your texts into your tape recorder for future listening is the best way to study. A tactile learner needs to spend extra time in the skill laboratory or at home practicing the skills step by step, preferably with a peer watching. Computer-based instruction may also assist this type of learner by allowing some tactile interaction during the lesson. The actual performance of skills and patient care in the clinical setting is the other major mode of learning available for a tactile learner. Elsevier's *Virtual Clinical Excursions*, geared to your textbook, incorporate visual, auditory, and kinesthetic learning.

Texts

Buy your required textbooks immediately. Put your name in them. When studying, remember to check each possible text that might contain information required for the next lecture day's topics. Text information changes very frequently in the health occupation field, and it is not a good idea to rely on a friend's old texts. The required textbooks are essential to your success. If you absolutely cannot afford a text right now, go to the library and see if there is a copy on reserve. Read the library copy, and make buying your own a high priority.

Reading

You will absorb more from your reading if you find a quiet place with few distractions in which to read. If you must read with other people's activity going on around you, consider masking the noise and distraction by using a pair of foam earplugs or earphones and a radio with soft music. Earplugs are available at pharmacies. Some students who are parents have found that it is best for them to go to bed with their children, get up in the middle of the night for a few hours to read and study, and then sleep a few more hours before the beginning of the day.

Reading should be done in an organized, consistent manner. **Unfamiliar words should be looked up** in the glossary of the text or the dictionary as they are encountered, and meanings should be jotted down. The SQ4R (survey, question, read, recite, record, review) study method is a popular method of tackling reading and study assignments used in many colleges and universities. Table 1-3 provides a synopsis of this method. It is described in greater length in various study skill books.

TABLE 1-3 SQ4R Study Method

	S	Survey	**R**	Recite
	Q	Question	**R**	Record (Write)
	R	Read	**R**	Review

Survey:	Look over the chapter, reading all the headings, captions under photographs and illustrations, charts, and graphs, plus the summary or last paragraph. This gives you the core ideas in the chapter.
Question:	Make a question out of each heading. This arouses curiosity and focuses on the content, and brings to mind information you already know.
Read:	Begin actively reading for an answer to the question. Read only one section and be certain you have answered the question before continuing. Highlight or underline the important points as you find them.
Recite:	After finishing each section, look away from the book and, using your own words, recite the answer to your question. If you can do this, you know what is in the book. If not, you need to reread and consider. Continue in this manner through the entire reading assignment. Write study notes for your objectives as you finish each section by either writing an answer to the objective, or by making an outline for the items listed in the content column of the syllabus.
Record (Write):	Record the information in some fashion. Use a highlighter to mark directly on the specific information in the text, take notes, or use a combination of the two. It is important to read and understand the material first, and then go back and record.
Review:	When you have finished the assignment for the next lecture session, look over your notes to understand the points and their relationships to each other. Check your memory by trying to answer each objective in the syllabus without looking at your notes.

Try it; if it does not suit your needs, check your college library and bookstore for study books containing other methods.

Reading is the key to establishing the base of knowledge needed to function as a nurse. If you can find time to **read full chapters** rather than just a few pages about a particular disease or problem, you will remember the information more easily and you will develop a fuller understanding of the body systems, how homeostasis is affected by diseases, and why particular nursing interventions are effective in a particular instance. Studying this way from the beginning of nursing school, when reading assignments tend to be less lengthy, makes the upper-level courses much easier because you already will have read much of the material to be covered.

Nursing texts are large and heavy. If you have time to study at work, consider tearing out chapters to take to work with you. Heavy books are difficult to carry around, but single chapters are easily portable. This may sound like heresy when you have been taught not to damage a book, but it is a practical solution. Just be certain you keep the chapters neatly filed for future review. Most nursing texts are outdated within 4 or 5 years, so keeping texts for reference during your future years of professional practice won't work.

Students who have difficulty reading because of dyslexia or visual problems should contact the Braille Institute Library. Recordings of various nursing texts are available on audiotape for students who qualify for the program. The institute will provide a tape player along with the tapes. The phone number is (800) 808-2555, and the address is 741 North Vermont Avenue, Los Angeles, CA 90029.

Note Taking

Two types of notes should be taken: study notes in preparation for lecture and class notes during lecture or laboratory. Preparation before class greatly enhances learning because the material covered in class is not being encountered for the very first time. **Repetition is essential to retention of information.** Familiarity with the topics to be covered in class allows you to follow the instructor's presentation by listening actively and adding to notes as needed. When you try to write down extensive notes during class, much of what the instructor is saying is missed.

Preparatory study notes can be made by outlining the material covered in required reading or by writing out concise answers to the objectives to be covered in the lecture for the day. In either event, the required reading is done first, with key concepts underlined or highlighted in the text, tables, charts, and illustrations, and when the reading is done, the study notes are made.

When writing study notes, use an organizational method that leaves room for the addition of information during the lecture. As study notes are enhanced during the lecture, they become class notes. Books on how to study, available from the library, present various methods for taking study notes. Two examples are given in Figure 1-4.

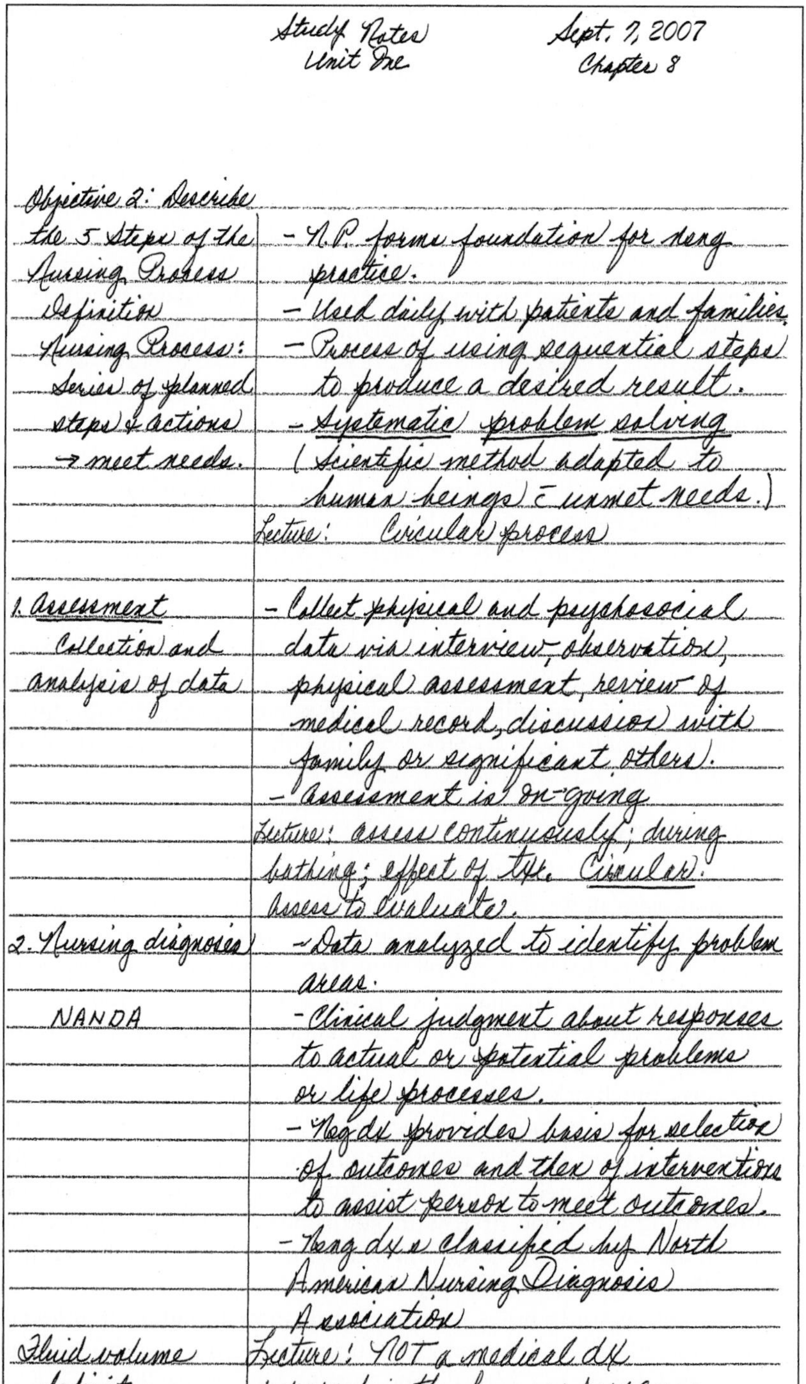

Study Notes   *Sept. 7, 2007*
Unit One   *Chapter 8*

Objective 2: Describe the 5 steps of the Nursing Process	– N.P. forms foundation for nsng practice.
Definition Nursing Process: Series of planned steps & actions → meet needs.	– Used daily with patients and families. – Process of using sequential steps to produce a desired result. – Systematic problem solving (Scientific method adapted to human beings c̄ unmet needs.) Lecture: Circular process
1. Assessment Collection and analysis of data	– Collect physical and psychosocial data via interview, observation, physical assessment, review of medical record, discussion with family or significant others). – assessment is on-going Lecture: assess continuously; during bathing; effect of txt. Circular: Assess to evaluate.
2. Nursing diagnosis NANDA	– Data analyzed to identify problem areas. – Clinical judgment about responses to actual or potential problems or life processes. – Nsg dx provides basis for selection of outcomes and then of interventions to assist person to meet outcomes. – Nsg dx classified by North American Nursing Diagnosis Association
Fluid volume deficit	Lecture: NOT a medical dx 1st part is the human response

FIGURE 1-4   Two examples of study note styles.

Study Notes Sept. 8, 2007
Chapter 8

Obj. 2 Describe the 5 steps of the nursing process

I. Nursing process	Lecture:
A. Foundation of practice	Circular, systematic
B. Used daily	process similar to
C. Sequential steps to-	scientific method.
ward desired result.	Use with every patient.
D. systematic problem	Core of professional
solving.	nursing. Methodical
	and orderly.
II. Assessment	Assessment is on-going.
A. Physical & psychosocial	Constantly assess - During
data gathered	bath & txs. Response to
1) patient	meds. Assess in order to
2) chart	evaluate. Use all senses.
3) family / s. o.	History taking via inter-
B. Analysis of data	view. Physical assessment
III. Nursing diagnosis	Data analyzed to find
A. Identify human	problem areas. Requires
response	clinical judgment.
B. Related factors	N orth
C. Pertinent defining	A merican
characteristics	N ursing
D. Choose from NANDA	Diagnoses
list.	Association
	Not a medical dx.
	Basis for choosing
	interventions to alleviate
	human response.

FIGURE **1-4,** cont'd.

It is also helpful to consider what would make a good exam question out of this material. What would you ask if you were the instructor? Jot down your ideas. After the exam on this material, go back and see how many of these questions were on the test.

Questions regarding unclear points should be jotted down during the preparation for class. However, it is wise to wait until the end of class to ask the questions because the instructor usually provides information during the class that will answer the questions.

The course outline or course syllabus should be consulted to identify material that will be covered during each class. Along with the required readings, the syllabus may also list other learning opportunities such as related periodical articles from professional nursing journals, audiovisual presentations available on campus, and computer learning modules available (see Figure 1-1). Whenever material is difficult to understand or unclear, using one or two of the other opportunities for learning can greatly increase comprehension and retention of the material. Well-written professional nursing journal articles are an invaluable resource. A bibliography or reference list for such articles is often included in the course outline or course syllabus. Check your college library's list of available journals. Use a computer and the Internet to connect to MEDLINE, CINAHL, and PsycINFO to search databases for appropriate articles in the journals available to you. Ask the college librarian to help if you are unfamiliar with accessing computerized databases. **It is a time-saving idea to subscribe immediately to at least one of the major professional nursing journals when you enter nursing school.** Reading a journal each month will add considerably to your knowledge base in nursing. *Nursing 2007, RN, Nursing Made Incredibly Easy*, and *American Journal of Nursing* are the four leading journals most useful to students. *Image* is the SNA journal and has articles that are geared particularly to students rather than practicing nurses.

Once study notes have been prepared and then converted to class notes, they should be reviewed as soon after class as possible. Once a week all of the study notes for the material covered that week should be reviewed. All notes for material to be covered on an exam should be reviewed in the few days preceding the test.

Tape-Recording Lectures. If you have difficulty following a particular instructor's presentation, or just don't seem to get all that is given in a lecture, the use of a tape recorder during class can be invaluable. However, the instructor's permission must be obtained before taping. It often has been said that the average student hears only 30% of what is said during a class period. Of course it is necessary to take time to review the tapes and add to your study notes as appropriate. Tapes can also be listened to in the car going back and forth to school and to work, thus increasing the actual study time for the student who must work many hours. You can use tapes while preparing meals, doing yard work, ironing, or performing other household chores that lend themselves to listening while doing.

Computer Skills. Honing your computer skills with a good grasp of Microsoft Office will make you a more efficient, and better organized, student. You will be expected to do research on the Internet either at home, at school, or on a library computer. Facility with a word processing program such as Microsoft Word will help you put together nursing care plans and written assignments quickly. As you progress through your nursing courses, creating nursing care plans on the computer can save you a lot of repetitive writing. With files of saved care plans, you can cut and paste, individualizing the new plan for a particular patient.

Excel is also a valuable program to learn. It is used in one way or another on almost any job these days. PowerPoint will most likely be needed for BSN students who are asked to do class presentations. This is the presentation software that is used throughout the business world. An e-mail program is valuable for contacting fellow students and instructors. It is also useful as a way for a busy nursing student to stay in touch with friends.

The Internet is a wonderful source for information on medical and nursing topics. Many materials are available to help you with patient teaching. Chat rooms especially for nurses or nursing students can help you get questions answered and provide a support group. Your school may have a bulletin board especially for its nursing students that features important announcements and reminders

You will be asked to do research, and the Internet has a wealth of information. It is essential to know how to evaluate the sites and information you find on the World Wide Web (Table 1-4). There are sites for students that can be helpful. Check out the Student Nurse Forum at http://kcsun3.tripod.com and the Allnurses.com student nurse page located at http://allnurses.com/Student_Nursing.

You should become familiar with the school intranet system where syllabi, class notes, instructions, announcements for class, and other information may be posted. The intranet platform that the school uses as the software shell, such as Blackboard, Web-CT, or E-College, should have a tutorial available to help you navigate the·site and areas within it you will need.

Study Groups

Depending on your learning style, you may find that joining a study group helps you prepare better for tests. The advantage of being in a study group is that you receive the benefit of the other members' viewpoints on topics and on what is most important in the material to be covered on a test. Some study groups divide up the objectives of a unit and each member prepares the answers to a certain number of the objectives. This works well if each member does a thorough job. However, some students cannot simply read and memorize material; they retain the

TABLE 1-4 Computer Competency Checklist for Taking Online Classes

You should know how to use:
▼ Microsoft Windows
▼ A word processing program such as Word
▼ Presentation software such as PowerPoint
▼ A spreadsheet such as Excel
▼ A database such as Access

You should be able to:
▼ Access an Internet service or Internet service provider, preferably high-speed
▼ Enable a firewall
▼ Use a virus protection program
▼ Install software programs
▼ Install plug-ins
▼ Format a floppy disk or save to a CD-ROM
▼ Download and save files
▼ Save a file of your work to your hard drive and to a disk or CD-ROM
▼ Copy, cut, and paste sections of text within a document and between documents
▼ Use an Internet search engine
▼ Perform searches for information and articles given a subject
▼ Reload a page in a Web browser
▼ Clear the cache or temporary Internet files in a Web browser

For accessing and handling e-mail, you should be able to:
▼ Set up an e-mail account with an Internet provider
▼ Send, receive, and open e-mail messages
▼ Open e-mail attachments
▼ Reply to e-mail messages
▼ Print e-mail messages
▼ Save e-mail to folders
▼ Attach files to e-mail messages
▼ Delete e-mail messages from the computer

---

information better if they write it out themselves. When looking for a study group, **remember that it is to your advantage to study with people who are more knowledgeable and who are getting as good or better grades than you are.**

When working with a study group, it is best to have done the reading and preparation for the material to be discussed before you meet. Discussion of the material will round out your knowledge of the subject, and hearing about it again will reinforce it in your memory.

Tutoring

Tutoring may be available on your campus for students who are not doing well. Check with the tutoring center, learning center, or learning resources center to see if this service is available. Look in the college handbook.

Often, this service is free to students and is provided by a higher-level student who has a high grade point average. Sometimes tutoring is available on a fee-for-service basis. The main point is to seek help as soon as you determine that you need it.

Taking an Online Course

When considering taking a class online, ask yourself if you are a self-motivator and are highly disciplined about schoolwork. Without face-to-face contact with a teacher, it is up to you to take more initiative in obtaining assignments, getting clarification when there are questions, and completing required work.

Before signing up for an online course, explore the course description and requirements. Be certain that the computer you will use meets the minimum specifications and that you have the required software installed. Make certain that the course will meet your needs, such as credit toward graduation, prerequisite credit for another course you will take later, or other requirements. If the class is offered by a different college than the one you are attending, be certain the credit will be transferable. Look at Table 1-4 to determine if your level of computer competence is sufficient to get you through the course.

Once you are enrolled, find out what the expectations of the student are. If they are not clear, e-mail the instructor and ask for the specific expectations. Consider the expectations and look at how your own strengths fit what is expected. Consider what challenges you will face in the course. Do you have the technical skills you will need? You should become familiar with the software platform that the college offering the course uses to present online courses (e.g., Blackboard, Web CT, E-College). Work through the tutorial offered by the college for the platform if you are unfamiliar with it. Increase your Internet search skills if you have not done a lot of academic searching. If in doubt about how to do this, check with your librarian or the computer lab personnel. They can point you to materials and tutorials that will be helpful. Review Table 1-5 on how to evaluate the content on a Web page.

Time management is extremely important when engaging in distance learning. If there are set times that the instructor will be available, plan your study time then so that if questions arise you might obtain an answer quickly. If there are set chat room times for communication with fellow students or the instructor, be online and available at those times. Write these times into your daily time map.

Most online classes are organized into a series of modules. Set up files for each module and keep everything pertaining to each module together. This way you will have everything ready when you work on a particular module. Accordion files are great for this purpose.

Be aware that Internet searches can be very time consuming and schedule enough time to do your research. Start your research well ahead of the time a paper or project is due. Check the class bulletin board daily for postings from faculty or students.

TABLE **1-5 Evaluating a Web Page**

▼ Who wrote the page? What are the person's qualifications and associations? Can you contact him or her?

▼ What institution publishes this piece? Check the domain of the document in the URL. (Preferred domains are .edu, .gov, .org, and .net.)

▼ When was the piece produced? Is it current and timely? Has it been updated since it was written?

▼ Is the information cited authentic (can you verify it with other sources)?

▼ What is the purpose of the piece?

▼ What is the point of view? What opinions are expressed by the author? Is bias evident? What is it?

▼ Is the piece written objectively?

▼ Could the piece be a spoof or ironic?

▼ Is there a way to satisfy questions or reservations you have about the piece?

▼ How up-to-date are links (if they are provided)?

Note that communication within an online course is slower than in the classroom. There will often be a delay between an e-mail question you send to the instructor and receipt of an answer. Whenever you don't understand something about an assignment or a reading, seek clarification from the instructor right away. Be patient when waiting for an answer; don't send repeated e-mails with the same questions.

Often an online course will require you to work as part of a group on a project. Try to balance your interaction so that you don't end up doing more than your share of the project. Keep communication open and timely between the group members so that progress on each part of the project will be evident. Because your grade depends on all the members of the group finishing their portion of the project, plan some extra time to help pick up the slack if someone doesn't come through with their part of the work.

Taking online classes can be a plus because they are more time-flexible than an on-campus class. You schedule when you will go online to do your class work. Some degree programs can be accomplished totally with online courses. (See Chapter 4.)

Doing Your Best on Tests

It's a good idea at the beginning of each week to scan your calendar in the *Student Planner* to check for the next test date. The best way to decrease test anxiety is to study the material sufficiently and get a good night's sleep before the examination. Last-minute cramming doesn't work for very many people.

Planning Your Preparation. When organizing to study specifically for an examination, review the instructor's designation of the material to be covered on this particular test. Do this at least a week before the test. Gather your study notes together: these should consist of the notes you took from your text readings, plus the lecture notes you added to these notes; or the written answers to the objectives to be included on the test, plus notes from the lecture. If time permits, consolidate your notes by making specific test notes from your study/class notes. On these sheets, put the data that you feel are most important in a concise form. Include material from special sources such as required films or articles. Review your concise test notes each night.

Divide up the material for the number of days you have before the test and systematically review your full notes at least once more. If time permits, you can go back and review what you have highlighted in your texts as well. If you belong to a study group, the day before the exam, meet and question each other on the objectives and what the group feels is the most important material, the material an instructor would most likely cover in an exam.

Day before the Exam. Review the syllabus or course outline of the material to be covered on the test. Read the content column, as well as the objectives, and review anything that you cannot immediately recall. Pay close attention to vocabulary and terms.

Night before the Exam. Get at least 7 hours of sleep. Eat a normal meal before going to school. If the test is late in the morning, take a high-powered snack with you to eat 20 minutes before the exam. The brain works best when it has the glucose necessary for cellular function. Stay away from other nervous students before the test. Stop reviewing at least 30 minutes before the exam; take a walk, go to the library and read a magazine, listen to music, or do something else relaxing. Go to the test room a few minutes before class time so that you are not rushed in settling down in your seat. Tune out what others are saying. Crowd tension is contagious, so stay away from it.

During the Exam. There are certain things that you can do to enhance your chance of success during a test. Suggestions include the following:

Multiple-Choice Tests

▼ Note the number of questions and the total time allotted for the test to determine at what time you should be halfway through the questions, and then note at what time you should be three-quarters of the way finished. Look at the clock only every 10 minutes or so. Plan to leave 5 to 10 minutes at the end of the test to check your work and your answer sheet.

▼ Read the preliminary instructions for taking the test very carefully. Check the chalkboard for notation of any changes or correction of printing errors.

▼ Calm yourself by taking time to close your eyes, put down your pencil, relax, and deep breathe for a few minutes to relax your body and relieve tension. Do this as needed if you feel especially tense during the exam.

▼ If you are allowed to write on the test booklet, underline all **pertinent** data and circle key words in the question.

▼ Cover the answers before you read the questions on multiple-choice tests. Read the question and think about what the answer should be, then see if such an answer is among the choices.

▼ For questions in which you need to "select all that apply," cover the answers while looking at the question stem and think about, or jot down, what fits. Then look at each of the choices and circle the number or letter of each choice that fits correctly with the question.

▼ For fill-in-the-blank questions, choose the word or words that immediately come to mind.

▼ Some questions will ask you to identify a spot on an anatomic model where you would do something or where something occurs. Locate the landmarks on the model carefully before indicating the correct spot.

▼ Eliminate wrong choices by marking through the letters or numbers of the choices.

▼ After choosing an answer, go back and reread the stem along with your chosen answer to it. Does it fit correctly? The choice that grammatically fits the stem and contains the correct information is the best choice.

▼ Don't read too much into the question. Stay away from the thought that it is a trick question. If you have nursing experience, ask yourself how a classmate who is inexperienced would answer this question just from what is in the textbooks and what has been given in the lectures.

▼ If you don't understand a question, raise your hand and ask the instructor. If there is a word in the question that you do not understand, raise your hand and ask for the meaning.

▼ Avoid choosing answers that use words such as *always, never, must, all, none,* and so forth. If you are confused about the question, read the choices, labeling them true or false, and choose the answer that is the odd one out (i.e., the one false one or the one true one). When a question is framed in the negative, such as "When assessing for pain, you should *not…*," the false option is the correct choice.

▼ Don't puzzle over any one question for too long. Skip it, and mark it to go back to when you have finished the other questions.

▼ Do keep track of the correlating question number on the Scantron answer sheet as you work through a multiple-choice test. Be careful when you skip a question also to skip the corresponding space on the Scantron sheet.

▼ Check your Scantron sheet to see that there are not two marks on any one line that would throw all the remaining answers off track of the correct question numbers.

▼ Choose the *best* answer for questions asking for a single answer. There may be more than one answer that is correct, but one answer may contain more information, or more important information, than another.

▼ When you are unsure of an answer, jot what you know about the topic in the margin without looking at the answers. Then look at the answers and follow your best instinct.

▼ **Never erase and change an answer** unless you read the question or the answer incorrectly or remembered a specific piece of information that has a bearing on the question. If you find you miss questions a lot because you erase answers, cut the eraser off the end of the pencil you take to the exam. If you find you have read a question wrong and really need to erase, raise your hand and ask the instructor for an eraser. This technique has helped numerous students raise their test grades considerably.

▼ At the end of the test, reread the questions, making certain you understood each one correctly. Check that the answer sheet is marked in the right location for each answer.

Essay Exams

▼ Divide your time according to the number of questions to be completed.

▼ Quickly outline the content of your answer before you begin writing.

▼ Answer the questions you know best first; it will help build your confidence.

▼ If you don't think you know the answer, take a bit of time to jot down everything you know about the *topic* of the question. Then try to formulate the answer.

▼ If you have absolutely no clue as to the answer of a question, try to think of something creative to write. Sometimes an instructor will give you a few points for your creativity. Anything is better than blank space on an essay exam.

▼ Reread each question and then read the answer you have written, making certain that it actually answers the question asked.

▼ Be certain your handwriting is legible.

▼ Pay attention to correct grammar, punctuation, and spelling.

NCLEX-RN®/NCLEX-PN® New Format Exam Questions

You may find that questions on your nursing exams are patterned after the NCLEX-PN® exam. There are four new types of questions on the exam.

1. Multiple-response, multiple-choice questions

Example: A client is prescribed a low-fat diet. In counseling him or her about food choices you would tell him or her to avoid: (Select all that apply.)

1. butter
2. barbequed ribs

3. grilled salmon
4. Caesar salad
5. hamburgers
6. whole milk
   Answer: 1, 2, 5, 6

2. Fill-in-the-blank questions
   Example: A client has an intravenous (IV) infusion ordered of D5 ½ NS 1000 mL at 100 mL/hr. If the IV tubing will deliver 15 drops per mL, the IV should be set to deliver _____ drops per minute.
   Answer: 25

3. Illustrated/graphic questions
   Example: You are performing a physical examination on a client. When listening to the heart, you would place your stethoscope over the apex to count the apical pulse. Indicate on the diagram the location of the apex of the heart. (Place the cursor over the correct area and click during the computerized NCLEX® examination.)
   Answer: c

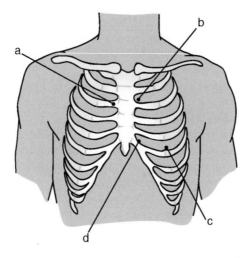

4. Prioritizing or sequencing questions
   Example: When catheterizing a female client, you would use sterile technique. Place the steps of the catheterization procedure in the correct sequence.
   1. Lubricate the catheter.
   2. Don sterile gloves.
   3. Cleanse the meatus.
   4. Drape the genital area.
   5. Locate the urinary meatus.
   6. Insert the catheter.
      Answer: 5, 4, 2, 3, 1, 6

There also will be NCLEX® examination questions in the traditional multiple-choice format with one correct answer.

Troubleshooting Your Exam Performance. If you are not achieving as high a score on tests as you feel you should, review the following questions to find ways in which you might improve your chance to score higher.

▼ How many hours per week are you spending in quality uninterrupted study time?

▼ How well can you concentrate during each segment of your study time? Are you too tired to concentrate?

▼ How many hours are you working? How many credit hours are you taking? Are there enough hours in the week to study adequately?

▼ Are you doing your reading before class? Are you reading whole chapters?

▼ Are you reading in each pertinent textbook? Fundamentals of nursing, medical-surgical nursing, pediatric nursing, obstetric nursing, nutrition, psychiatric nursing, pharmacology, and so forth?

▼ How do you go about beginning a unit of study? Do you review the pertinent anatomy and physiology before beginning the text readings if you do not remember it?

▼ Do you study the objectives in the syllabus, including the topics in the content column, as you go?

▼ Do you take study notes after you have first read the material and before a lecture in a format that allows you to add lecture notes to your study notes?

▼ Do you use a tape recorder in class? Do you review the tapes?

▼ Do you have more than normal test anxiety? Have you worked with a counselor on this? Have you practiced suggested relaxation and confidence-building techniques regularly?

▼ Do you review each day's lecture notes that night?

▼ Are you using good test-taking techniques?
  ▼ Underlining key words in the stem and choices
  ▼ Eliminating wrong choices
  ▼ After choosing an answer, checking that it fits with the stem and that it answers the question asked
  ▼ Using test time evenly
  ▼ Refraining from erasing and changing answers frequently

▼ Do you have a regular study group or study partner? Are the others in the group doing well? (If not, study with someone who is!)

▼ Are you relying on reading in a review book to get you through instead of reading in your texts? Are you relying on reading in a review book before tests instead of studying your own notes?

Find your problem areas and remedy them, and your test scores will improve. Students often feel that they are studying a lot, but they are studying at home with constant interruptions to their concentration. Going to the neighborhood library to study is one option. Organizing to study during the day when roommates, partners, and children are out of the house, and then doing chores, shopping, laundry, and errands at night, is another alternative.

Problems with success at school should be remedied as soon as they are identified. Many students go along thinking things will get better without taking any initiative to make certain that things do get better. Too often, students wait until they are in serious trouble with poor grades before changing study habits or number of work hours. You've invested a lot in your education; guard that investment by giving yourself the best chance for success.

Taking the NCLEX® Examination

During your final semester of the nursing program, you will receive information from your instructors on the mechanics of signing up to take the NCLEX® examination. The test is taken on a computer at a designated testing site. After you graduate from your nursing program and have met the educational requirements for licensure, you will receive a ticket that allows you to sit for the NCLEX-RN® or NCLEX-PN® examination, depending on which type of program you complete. The exams are offered four times a year and are available across the United States. Each person may take the exam three times within a 12-month period but must wait 90 days before retaking the exam. The exam may be taken in any state, but licensure will be issued by the state in which you reside. Visit www.ncsbn.com on the Internet for the test plan and a variety of resources to help you prepare for the exam. This Web site will also provide a list of states that have a reciprocity compact agreement for licensure (where license is obtained in one state, but is also valid in another state).

Obtaining Licensure

After passing the NCLEX-PN® or NCLEX-RN® examination you will receive a licensure ticket from the testing center. That ticket, along with the paperwork from your school documenting completion of the required courses and clinical hours, must be submitted along with the application for licensure to your state board of nurse examiners.

There are specific regulations and requirements for any person who has had a criminal conviction or been treated for a psychiatric occurrence. **It is wise to check with your state board of nursing before beginning the nursing program or during the first course to obtain these regulations and requirements.**

2

Getting the Most out of the Clinical Experience

APPROACHING THE CLINICAL EXPERIENCE

You may be assigned to various clinical facilities during the semester. Clinical locations are usually at hospitals, long-term care facilities, home health agencies, community clinics, psychiatric outpatient clinics, day care centers, or school clinics. At some of these facilities you may be an observer rather than a care provider. Your instructor will clarify how you should prepare for the type of clinical facility to which you are assigned.

It is normal to be concerned and apprehensive about your first contact with a patient. Be assured that you will not be required to do more for that patient than your nursing course has prepared you to do. Remember that there is always a staff nurse assigned to that patient as well. It is usual for the student to prepare at school for skills to be performed in clinical and to be evaluated on critical skills by an instructor. Only then is the student expected to apply those skills with real patients. Critical skills are those in which accuracy is of vital importance to the patient's treatment (such as taking vital signs) or those that are invasive and have a potential for injury to the patient (such as giving an injection or inserting a urinary catheter).

Most students fear hurting the patient. The best way to prevent this is to be as prepared as possible for the clinical patient assignment and to refuse to perform tasks for which instruction and verification of correct technique by an instructor have not yet occurred. Tell the nurse in charge of the patient that you may not perform the skill or care involved if you have not covered it at school.

Preparing for Clinical Patient Care

At some schools, instructors assign patients to the students; other schools require that each student choose patients for the clinical assignment. Either way, you will have some pertinent information ahead of time. You will know the patient's diagnosis, what treatments are scheduled, any tests the patient may have that day, the names of the medications, and the patient's age and sex before you see the patient. If specific patients can't be assigned the day before the clinical experience, you will know the type of unit on which the patient assignment will be located. If you are able to choose your own patient assignment, do a quick review of each patient's chart when obtaining your information (Table 2-1).

TABLE 2-1 Quick Chart Review

Sheet	Information
Face sheet	Marital status, age, insurance coverage, occupation, significant others, religion, location of home
Physician's order sheet	Tests ordered, medications, intravenous solutions, treatments to be done (admitting day up to today)
Physician's history	Overview of total health status and summary of current and physical health problems; allergies
Physician's progress notes	Gives clues to future tests and orders; status of problems
Nursing admission assessment	Medications and supplements taken at home, allergies; prosthetic devices such as hearing aid, glasses; previous health problems and hospitalizations; previous surgeries; and so forth
Laboratory reports	Tests that have been completed, results, and any abnormal values
Other test results	Findings that are abnormal (read the conclusions); pathology reports tell whether patient has cancer
Medication sheets	Medications ordered; how often patient is taking as-needed (PRN) medications and what they are
Consultation sheets	Conclusions of other members of the health care team
Nurse's notes	Care given for previous 24 hours; problems encountered; changes in plan of care; visitors; psychologic outlook
Flow sheets and electronic patient record (EPR)	Vital signs, intake and output, intravenous fluids, blood administered, neurologic signs and changes, and so forth
Nursing care plan, collaborative care plan, care pathway, or "needs" list	Lists the problems or nursing diagnoses, with goals and care interventions to be done
Operative report	Conclusion tells what was done; abnormalities found and problems encountered; amount of blood loss

Also ask to see the patient care card, Kardex plan, or computer patient care sheets. These provide directions for everything that the nurse should be doing for the patient. Look for the nursing care plan in the chart or the "needs" list; it will give you some ideas about the patients' nursing problems and actual nursing diagnoses. Be certain to check with the nurse in charge so you will know which patients other students have already chosen before selecting your assignment.

Preparation for clinical patient care involves reading about the disease process or problem and noting the following:

▼ Causes and contributing factors (etiology)
▼ Usual signs and symptoms of the disorder

▼ Common medical treatment for the disorder, including medications
▼ Common nursing problems or nursing diagnoses the patient is likely to have
▼ Psychosocial ramifications

If you do not receive a specific patient assignment before clinical, find out what unit you will be on and determine the types of patients usually cared for on that unit. Then read about those types of patients. For example, if you are assigned to an orthopedic unit, you should read about fractures, traction, back problems, and hip and knee replacements. When assigned to a general surgical unit, review preoperative and postoperative care, dressing changes, nasogastric suction, care of wound suction devices, catheters, and so forth. The section in your textbook relative to the type of hospital unit you will be working on will give you some clues as to the information you will need. An Internet search can usually provide information on the disease condition and appropriate teaching. Search by subject or enter a medical site such as those listed in Chapter 6, "Obtaining Information Via the Internet." If you don't have your own computer, use the school computer or go to the school or public library to gain access.

Reviewing Skills for Patient Care

Next, information should be reviewed about the treatments to be done such as dressing changes, maintaining traction, hot or cold applications, intravenous (IV) therapy, and the like. You should review each treatment even if it is not a task you are currently capable of doing. Clinical learning takes place when you are prepared and observe an experienced nurse perform the skill. Of course, as each nursing course progresses, you will be prepared to perform more of the skills. Instructors generally require that the student review a skill just before performing it in the clinical area.

When on the nursing unit, you can look up the skill or treatment in the procedure manual kept on the floor. Each nursing unit should have this manual available to staff. It gives the specific steps and protocol for doing each nursing procedure. To be within safe, legal boundaries, each nurse should perform the designated procedure in the manner described. It is up to the student to seek experience in performing skills. Choose patients for your assignment who require some skills you can perform. During report, mention that when your assigned work is done, you would like to perform other tasks for which you are prepared. Be specific about what you are looking for—injections, catheterizations, IV therapy experience, and so forth.

Looking up Medications

From clinical day 1, you should look up each medication your assigned patients are receiving. Although students do not usually give medication during the first weeks of the first nursing course, there are thousands of medications in use today, and the best way to learn about them is to attach a patient situation to the medication. Besides, even if you are not giving the medication, you will be expected to watch for possible side effects of the various drugs the patient is receiving. **You are legally liable** if you cause harm to a patient from a medication you have administered.

Drug Text or Handbook. If you have a pharmacology text, look up and review the information on medications. If you don't have such a text, you may wish to purchase a drug reference written especially for nurses—*2007 Mosby's Drug Consult for Nurses,* for example. There are many such books on the market, and your school bookstore probably stocks a variety. Information you want includes the following:

▼ Classification of the drug (antibiotic, antihypertensive, etc.)
▼ What it's supposed to do (its action in understandable terms)
▼ Usual dosage and route of administration
▼ Potential serious adverse effects
▼ Common side effects
▼ Drug interactions
▼ Special nursing implications, such as whether it needs to be given with food or an hour after meals, whether sunlight should be avoided, and so forth

To prevent fear of making a medication error, review the Safety Guidelines to Prevent Medication Errors in Chapter 5.

As you progress through your nursing courses, it will become more apparent that if you understand how a drug works, you will be able to determine easily what the possible side effects and nursing implications are.

The student who is well prepared for each clinical experience will be less anxious, will function in the clinical setting more efficiently, will have less fear of hurting a patient, and will learn more.

Nursing Care Plans

After orientation you probably will be required to bring a written nursing care plan or care map for each clinical day. Some schools require a certain number of nursing diagnoses or problems to be worked out; others want a complete care plan for each patient. From the data gathering you did for your assignment, you will have the patient's medical diagnoses, diagnostic test data, some history, and the nursing diagnoses that were listed in the chart. Analyze your data and determine your own nursing diagnoses as you have been taught to do in your fundamentals of nursing course in the unit on nursing process. Practical nursing (licensed practical nurse/licensed vocational nurse [LPN/LVN]) students may be given the patient's nursing diagnoses and asked to construct a plan from that point. Each nursing diagnosis must be correlated with supporting data. Determine appropriate goals or outcome criteria for each diagnosis. Ask yourself if the expected outcome you have written is measurable: Will you be able to tell from evaluation data whether it has been met? Read your textbooks for ideas about actions that are appropriate to meet the patient's needs for each nursing diagnosis. For example, if the diagnosis is "Risk for Infection related to poor nutritional status," then, in addition to monitoring for signs of infection such as increased temperature, increased white blood cell count, redness, pain and swelling of the wound, or purulent drainage, you would include actions to improve nutritional status. Such actions would be to increase protein and vitamin C intake and encourage a well-balanced diet with sufficient fluids and calories to maintain a positive nutritional balance. Of course, using good handwashing and aseptic technique for dressing changes and employing standard precautions are included as well. Actions must be individualized for each patient; actions for the patient who is diabetic would be a little different than those for another patient. When writing nursing care plans, you must pull together information you have learned from anatomy and physiology, microbiology, psychology, and your nursing courses and apply it to a particular situation. Your text for fundamentals of nursing plus the text for the specific clinical area you are assigned to (obstetrics, medical or surgical floor, pediatrics, or psychiatric area) will provide information for usual nursing diagnoses and actions for patients with the medical diagnosis or problems your patients have.

Nursing Diagnoses. There are many nursing care plan books on the market to help you. They are handy in that they sum up the generalities of nursing diagnoses and actions for a particular disorder. Your school bookstore probably stocks several of these volumes. Choose one that is easy to understand and that is as close to the format your school uses as possible. Be aware though that you still must individualize the care plans for your patients. Many have the care plans on a CD-ROM so that you can individualize them for your patients on the computer. Read through the plan listed and ask yourself if each item applies to your specific patient before including it on your own nursing care plan. Nursing care planning is a thinking process, not just a copying process. The whole idea is to systematically devise a plan to meet the patient's basic needs. It is best to look at patients holistically, including psychosocial needs, as well as physical needs. One way to check yourself when writing care plans is to see if you have covered all areas of basic need. Table 2-2 presents a checklist using the acronym RN'S HOPE to be sure that you have considered all areas. **Two nursing diagnoses that students often overlook are "Self-Care Deficit" and "Deficient Knowledge."**

Each instructor views nursing care plans a bit differently, even within a particular school of nursing. Get to know what your instructor wants and how things should be worded in general. Ask to see an example of a nursing care plan that the instructor thinks is very good.

Rationales. Many schools require a scientific rationale or principle for each action you list on your care plan. What is desired is a *scientifically based* reason the action works. An example for interventions included in the Sample Nursing Care Plan (Figure 2-1) is *Intervention:* Discourage

Text continued on p. 36

TABLE 2-2 Choosing Nursing Diagnoses

Once you have analyzed your assessment data and chosen the most obvious nursing diagnoses for your patient's nursing care plan, you should review each area of possible need to make certain that you have not missed an important area. One way to do this is to keep in mind the acronym RN'S HOPE, which covers all areas of basic needs:

R   Rest and activity needs
N   Nutritional needs
S   Safety needs
H   Hygiene needs
O   Oxygenation needs
P   Psychosocial needs
E   Elimination and education needs

Examples of nursing diagnoses grouped for problems for each area of basic need include the following:

Rest and Activity
Activity intolerance
Impaired physical mobility
Fatigue
Disturbed sleep pattern
Pain, acute or chronic

Nutrition
Risk for impaired liver function*
Imbalanced nutrition: less than body requirements
Imbalanced nutrition: more than body requirements
Feeding self-care deficit
Risk for unstable glucose level*
Impaired swallowing
Deficient fluid volume or excess
Nausea

Safety
Risk for acute confusion*
Contamination*
Risk for contamination*
Readiness for enhanced comfort*
Readiness for enhanced immunization status*
Risk for injury
Impaired physical mobility
Risk for infection
Impaired skin integrity
Risk for impaired skin integrity
Disturbed sensory perception
Disturbed thought processes
Impaired verbal communication
Hyperthermia
Hypothermia
Risk for falls
Impaired memory
Wandering

TABLE 2-2 Choosing Nursing Diagnoses—cont'd

Hygiene
Readiness for enhanced self-care*
Self-care deficit, toileting
Dressing/grooming
Self-care deficit
Impaired oral mucous membrane

Oxygenation
Ineffective airway clearance
Risk for aspiration
Ineffective breathing pattern
Impaired gas exchange
Ineffective tissue perfusion
Decreased cardiac output

Psychosocial
Ineffective coping
Readiness for enhanced decision-making*
Risk for compromised human dignity*
Interrupted family processes
Fear
Anxiety
Disturbed body image
Ineffective health maintenance
Impaired home maintenance
Readiness for enhanced hope*
Moral distress*
Readiness for enhanced power*
Chronic low self-esteem
Spiritual distress
Social isolation
Stress overload*

Elimination and Education
Constipation
Urinary incontinence, overflow*
Urinary incontinence, stress
Diarrhea
Bowel incontinence
Self-care deficit, toileting
Excess fluid volume
Sexual dysfunction
Deficient knowledge

*2006 additions.

The full North American Nursing Diagnosis Association (NANDA) list of accepted nursing diagnoses presents other possibilities. Remember that many nursing actions are used to prevent problems, and in this event these actions are grouped under a "risk for" nursing diagnosis. The three areas students most often overlook are self-care deficit, deficient knowledge, and the major reason the patient is in the hospital, such as fractured hip (impaired physical mobility) or myocardial infarction (decreased cardiac output).

In addition, **each medication to be administered and each procedure to be done should fit under some nursing diagnosis on the care plan as an intervention.**

Sample Nursing Care Plan

Selected nursing diagnoses, goals/expected outcomes, nursing interventions, and evaluations for a patient with hypertension

Situation: 53-year-old male with a blood pressure of 170/100 found during routine screening of all employees at a local plant. A visit to the hypertension clinic reveals that he is hypertensive, is 75 pounds overweight, smokes two packs of cigarettes a day, and eats snacks during the day and in the evening while watching television. The physician prescribes a low-sodium diet and a mild antihypertensive. During her interview with the patient, the nurse notes that he does not understand the nature of his illness, how his lifestyle is related to hypertension, and the purpose of the low-sodium diet and the expected action of the diuretic.

Nursing Diagnosis	Goals/Expected Outcome	Nursing Interventions	Evaluation
Ineffective tissue perfusion related to increased peripheral vascular resistance *SUPPORTING DATA* BP, 172/102; P, 96; feet cool and pale; pedal pulses, 1+; capillary refill > 4s.	Patient will maintain adequate tissue perfusion as evidenced by: 1. BP within normal limits at end of 3 weeks. 2. Pulse returns to normal range within 4 weeks. 3. Skin of feet warm and dry within 4 weeks. 4. Capillary refill time less than 3 sec within 4 weeks. Patient will quit smoking within 1 month.	Teach to take antihypertensive as ordered; and monitor BP b.i.d. Assess skin and peripheral pulses each visit. Discourage smoking; encourage him to quit smoking. Discourage intake of foods high in caffeine. Maintain sodium restrictions. Have patient weigh himself daily and keep record.	BP, 156/96; P, 86; skin on feet pale and cool; smoked only five cigarettes today; weight down 2 lb. Continue plan.
Imbalanced nutrition, more than body requirements related to overeating and lack of exercise *SUPPORTING DATA* Weight, 285 lbs; height, 6 ft; consumes lots of junk food between meals; no daily exercise program; watches television a lot.	Patient will lose 2 lbs within 2 months. Consultation with dietitian within 2 weeks. Patient will maintain 2-lb/wk weight loss until normal weight of 210 lbs is attained. Patient will have developed daily exercise plan within 2 weeks.	Explain need to lose excess weight; encourage him to participate in weight loss plan. Assist with development of daily exercise plan. Ask for dietary consult.	Weight, 283 lbs; is considering options for daily exercise plan.

Sample Nursing Care Plan—cont'd

Nursing Diagnosis	Goals/Expected Outcome	Nursing Interventions	Evaluation
Deficient knowledge related to self-care aspects of hypertension: how to take blood pressure, medication rationale and side effects, low-sodium diet, need for exercise, need for continued medical follow-up *SUPPORTING DATA* Does not know how to take blood pressure; has never taken anti-hypertensive medication; unaware of sodium content of foods and sodium's relationship to hypertension; unaware of the benefits of exercise on the cardiovascular system; complains of cost of going to doctor for a check-up.	Patient will demonstrate correct technique for taking own blood pressure within 1 week of teaching. Patient will explain action of antihypertensive medication and possible side effects 1 week after teaching session. Patient will describe effects of exercise on cardiovascular system after teaching session. Patient will state which foods are high in sodium when given a list from which to choose foods after teaching session. Before discharge patient will give three reasons why continued follow-up is necessary for patients with hypertension.	Develop teaching plan covering the following points: 1. How to take own blood pressure. 2. Action and side effects of antihypertensive medication. 3. Beneficial effects of exercise program on cardiovascular system. 4. How sodium increases water retention and elevates blood pressure. 5. Foods to avoid that contain excess sodium. 6. Potential complications of uncontrolled blood pressure and reasons for physician examination to detect beginning complications.	First teaching session completed; verbalizes action and three side effects of antihypertensive medication; can pick foods high in sodium from a list. Continue teaching and plan. Progressing toward outcomes.
Risk for ineffective coping related to lack of desire to quit smoking, even though he is hypertensive. *SUPPORTING DATA* States that he does not wish to quit smoking and doesn't really see the need to do so. All of his friends smoke.	Patient will verbalize how smoking affects the blood vessels 3 days after teaching session. Patient will verbalize desire to quit smoking within 1 month. Patient will institute a "no smoking" program within 1 month.	Teach how nicotine constricts the blood vessels, elevating blood pressure and decreasing blood flow to the periphery of the body. Encourage patient to quit smoking. Obtain American Heart Association, American Lung Association, and American Cancer Society materials regarding the dangers of smoking. Familiarize the patient with available community "Quit Smoking" programs. Encourage him to join support group for those who are quitting smoking.	Discussed effect of smoking on vessels; gave patient AHA materials to read; encouraged him to quit smoking; scheduled another session tomorrow. Continue plan.

FIGURE 2-1 Sample nursing care plan.

intake of foods high in caffeine. *Rationale:* The chemical caffeine causes blood vessels to constrict, which increases blood pressure.

The evaluation section of the nursing process cannot be completed until you carry out your plan of care during clinical hours. After you have cared for the patient, go back and revise your preliminary plan.

Some of the nursing diagnoses you listed may not be pertinent, and you may have discovered other problems and concerns that are more important to the patient. Delete actions that are ineffective and devise new ones to help meet your stated expected outcomes. Usually the care plan does not have to be recopied; you just add to it, perhaps in a different color ink to show what has been changed and updated.

Pathophysiology Statement. Some schools also require a pathophysiology statement concerning the patient's medical diagnosis or problem.

TABLE 2-3 Examples of Pathophysiology Statements

A pathophysiology statement usually consists of the etiology of the disease or disorder, the usual signs and symptoms compared with the individual patient's signs and symptoms, the usual treatment, and potential complications.

Example I
Cholelithiasis
Cholelithiasis is the presence of gallstones in the biliary system. They may be located in the gallbladder, the common duct, or the hepatic ducts of the liver. The stones may consist of cholesterol, pigments (mainly unconjugated bilirubin), or a combination of these substances with calcium carbonate, phosphate, or bile salts. Gallstones occur more frequently in women, and the incidence increases with age. This patient has the following risk factors: obesity, diabetes mellitus.

Usual signs and symptoms include pain, often in the upper right quadrant; jaundice; nausea and vomiting; bloating and indigestion; fatty food intolerance. This patient has upper midline pain radiating to the right shoulder blade, nausea, and intolerance to fatty foods.

Treatment consists of removing the stones surgically or breaking the stones up with lithotripsy or by chemical dissolution. This patient underwent laparoscopic cholecystectomy.

Complications include residual stones in a duct causing blockage, infection from the surgical procedure, and internal bleeding from surgery.

Example II
Myocardial Infarction
Atherosclerosis → coronary thrombosis (or embolus) → occlusion of artery→↓
   myocardial tissue perfusion → impaired muscle function →↓ cardiac output*
Potential complications include the following:
Necrosis of tissue
Dysrhythmia
Congestive heart failure
Death

*Can be done in the form of a concept map.

For beginning courses, a simple explanation of the diagnosis, including the physiologic changes the disease or disorder is causing and the signs and symptoms expected, usually is all that is necessary. **If the patient is undergoing or has undergone surgery, do the pathophysiology statement on the disorder that necessitated the surgery.** Include the type of surgical procedure performed and physiologic changes that the patient has experienced.

In more advanced courses, you should consider the course of the disease or disorder and the prognosis if there is no intervention. Determine what the potential complications of the disorder might be and discuss the effect of the problem on the patient's basic needs. Table 2-3 provides two examples of pathophysiology statements.

Writing pathophysiology statements helps you understand what is going on physiologically in the patient, and how that is causing interference with the patient's ability to provide for his or her own basic needs. That is where you put your nursing actions to work—you assist the patient in meeting basic needs when he or she is unable to do so. You attempt to prevent complications that would extend the illness or delay the surgical recovery.

Together your chart review, preparatory reading, pathophysiology statement, and construction of the preliminary nursing care plan have prepared you with most of the data you need to care adequately for your patient. You will add information from a shift report to help determine what care your patient will need that day.

Shift Report: What to Listen for

When listening to the morning/evening report, you should write down on your work organization sheet pertinent information about your patients and all nursing care to be done. Table 2-4 lists the information to be obtained.

If there was something you didn't understand, ask the nurse in charge about it. Verify with the staff nurse who is assigned to your patient your understanding of what you are responsible for in the care of the patient, and **state those tasks that are beyond your skill level.** Make certain that the staff nurse understands that you do not do tasks or assessments beyond your skill level. **This is your responsibility.** Nurses work with students from different schools and different course levels. Unless you state differently, the nurse may assume you are doing everything that needs to be done for the patient, and vital assessments and treatments may go undone.

Preparing for Patient Teaching

From the patient assignment information and through your reading about the disease process and nursing care, you will have an idea of areas in which patient teaching may be required. If the patient is having a diagnostic test done, read about the test and especially note the pretest and posttest nursing care. Consider what the patient might experience during the test. This will give you an edge in answering patient questions and help you know what to expect during your time of care. Having this information also helps with clinical time organization.

TABLE 2-4 Information to Obtain during Report

Room number and bed designation
Date of admission and physician
Diagnoses
Current surgery or delivery and type: vaginal or C-section; gravida; para
Surgery or tests scheduled for next 24 hours
Vital signs schedule   Neurologic signs schedule
Abnormalities to report to physician
Diet: NPO   I&O previous shift
Dextrose sticks   Insulin orders
Tubes: NG   Foley   Drains
Oxygen: Cannula   Mask   Flow rate   PRN   Continuous
IV location, type, when inserted   Solution hanging and amount left to count
          Solution to follow
Equipment: Fetal monitor   SCD   CPM   Traction/type
          PCA   Oximeter
Telemetry   Other
Treatments: Heat lamp   Sitz   Dressing changes   ROM
          TCDB   Spirometer   Heat/cold   K-pad
Type of bath: Shower   Assist   Complete bed bath
Activity: OOB   BSC   BRP   BRP with assistance
          Bed rest
PRN medications given last shift
Pain level
Impairments: Vision   Hearing   Paresis   Paralysis
          Amputation (old/new)
Mental status: Alert   Confused   Comatose
Medication changes
Problems
Concerns/need for order changes
Needed teaching
Psychosocial status
Patient-family dynamics
Amount of assistance needed

BRP, Bathroom priveleges; *BSC,* bedside commode; *CPM,* continuous passive motion; *I&O,* intake and output; *IV,* intravenous; *NG,* nasogastric; *NPO,* nothing by mouth; *OOB,* out of bed; *PCA,* patient-controlled analgesia; *PRN,* as needed; *ROM,* range of motion; *SCD,* sequential compression device; *TCDB,* turn, cough, and deep breathe.

Other areas in which teaching may be necessary include self-care tasks such as cast care, dressing changes at home, diabetic self-care, medication administration, preoperative teaching, and any other health care–related task the patient and family will be doing at home. Teaching for home care should begin early in the hospitalization. Useful materials for patient teaching can be found on the Internet. Search by topic or go to one of the medical sites listed in Chapter 6. Sometimes there will be useful diagrams or sets of instructions for self-care that are handy to give to the patient.

TABLE 2-5 Checklist for Discharge Teaching

Instructions must be given to each patient before discharge covering the following topics:

▼ Medications: name, dosage, times to be taken, special instructions
▼ Diet: what to eat, foods to avoid
▼ Activity: exercise, rest, lifting, stair climbing, driving, resumption of sexual activity; special instructions for use of crutches, cane, walker
▼ Breathing exercises: deep breathing and coughing schedule or schedule for incentive spirometry
▼ Wound care: how to cleanse; how to change the dressing; signs and symptoms to report
▼ Bathing: type of bath or shower permitted
▼ Next contact with the physician: when to call for appointment or time of appointment
▼ General instructions: report temperature more than 100.1° F, increase in pain, nausea and vomiting; and particular instructions for individual patient
▼ Special instructions: any specific points necessary for proper self-care

Provide written instructions whenever possible in addition to verbal instructions.

Every patient must receive discharge teaching and instructions before being released from the hospital. The topics covered are essentially the same for each patient, but the amount of instruction and the variations in care necessary at home depend on the patient's diagnosis or problem. Table 2-5 presents a checklist for discharge teaching so you can be prepared if your patient is released on your clinical day.

Work Organization

Regardless of the number of patients you are taking care of, organize your workday. Decide what you are going to do at which times based on the priority of the tasks. Shift report has given you data about when various things must be done. Vital signs are usually done at 8:00 AM, 12:00 PM (noon), 4:00 PM, and 8:00 PM. If treatments are scheduled bid (twice a day) or tid (three times a day), you have some leeway in deciding when you wish them to be done (whether you can do them or not—consult your staff nurse). Consider whether the patient will be having physical therapy or special tests. Will that mean he or she will be off of the unit for a while? Ask your staff nurse. Plan what time you will bathe the patient, make the bed, and do your more complete physical assessment. When will you do the dressing change or ambulate the patient? Plan time for turning, deep breathing, and coughing. Provide periods when the patient can rest. If you have several patients, plan your tasks in rotation so no one is neglected. Each patient should be seen at least every hour during the day shift. Initially you will probably be assigned to only one patient, but by the end of the first semester you should be caring for at least two.

Figure 2-2 provides a sample work organization plan. Figure 2-3 is a blank form that you may copy and use in clinical. A well-done work

Text continued on p. 44

SHIFT WORK ORGANIZATION SHEET

PATIENT/ROOM	8:00	9:00	10:00	11:00	12:00	13:00	14:00	15:00
J.D. 521	V.S. Quick Assess	9 30 Shower 9 45 Adressing		Full Assess Chart	V.S. Glucometer	Pre-op teaching Chart	I + O Tape report	Close chart
R.S. 523¹	V.S. 8 20 Quick Assess √IV	Feed Full Assess √IV	Bathe + Bed	Chart	Feed	Let Nap	Empty Foley I + O	Close chart
B.W. 523²	V.S. Quick Assess √IV	Full Assess √IV	Shower + Bed √IV	Chart √IV	V.S. √IV	√IV	I + O √IV	Close chart √IV
PATIENT/ROOM								

FIGURE 2-2 Sample shift work organization sheet.

MEDICATION TIMES

PATIENT/ROOM	7:30	8:00	9:00	10:00	11:00	12:00	13:00	14:00	15:00	PRN
J.D. 521	Insulin	✓✓	✓✓ ✓✓			S.S. Insulin		✓		Pain 10⁴⁰ 14¹⁰
R.S. 523¹			✓✓				✓✓			
B.W. 523²		✓	✓✓✓				✓			
PATIENT/ROOM										

FIGURE 2-2, cont'd.

SHIFT WORK ORGANIZATION SHEET

PATIENT/ROOM	8:00	9:00	10:00	11:00	12:00	13:00	14:00	15:00
PATIENT/ROOM								
PATIENT/ROOM								
PATIENT/ROOM								
PATIENT/ROOM								

FIGURE 2-3   Blank shift work organization sheet.

MEDICATION TIMES

PATIENT/ROOM	7:30	8:00	9:00	10:00	11:00	12:00	13:00	14:00	15:00	PRN
PATIENT/ROOM										
PATIENT/ROOM										
PATIENT/ROOM										
PATIENT/ROOM										

FIGURE 2-3, cont'd.

organization form provides a good guide by which to do your charting. At the end of each clinical day, review your work organization form to determine whether your plan worked. If it did not, think about what to change before you use the form again. Figure 2-4 is a sample of a patient care worksheet similar to that used by many nurses to jot down information during report.

HIPAA Requirements for Confidentiality. The federal privacy regulations came into effect April 2003. The privacy rules are part of the overall Health Insurance Portability and Accountability Act (HIPAA). The rules govern how client information is conveyed, stored, and shared. Table 2-6 presents a synopsis of the major points. **As a student you must not discuss anything about your patients/clients with anyone who is not directly involved in their care.** Refrain from talking about your patients with other students assigned to the same unit in the elevators or the cafeteria, where you may be overheard. If you are documenting via computer, do not leave the screen unattended while a patient record is viewable on it. Refrain from writing patient names on your written work; use only initials. When performing patient teaching or answering questions, keep your voice low and provide as much privacy as possible. Do not let

---

TABLE 2-6 Rights Provided by the Health Insurance Portability and Accountability Act (HIPAA)

HIPAA covers six patient rights and provider responsibilities:

Consent—Written consents must contain a clause that says the patient agrees to allow the provider to use and disclose his or her information for treatment, payment, and health care operations. A notice must be attached to the consent form.

Notice—The provider's obligations are outlined regarding the privacy of the patient's health care information. It includes the six patient rights and responsibilities of the provider. It details how the patient information will be protected and a process for filing a complaint if the patient believes privacy rights have been violated.

Access—The patient has the right to inspect and copy his or her medical record.

Amendment—A patient has the right to amend his or her record for the purpose of accuracy.

Accounting for disclosures—Providers are held accountable for how patients' medical information is handled. Tracking of any disclosures of information not related to treatment, payment, or health care operations, or that were not authorized by the patient, must occur.

Restriction of disclosure—The patient can request that the provider restrict the use and disclosure of his or her information. The provider does not, however, have to grant the request.

From deWit SC: *Fundamental concepts and skills for nursing*, ed 2, Philadelphia, 2005, Elsevier, p 32.

PATIENT CARE WORKSHEET

PATIENT	ROOM #	DIAGNOSIS	V/S	DIET	I & O	ACTIVITY	MISC.

FIGURE 2-4   Patient care worksheet.

anyone not directly involved in the patient's care view the medical record. HIPAA gives patients the right to correct erroneous information in their records and the right to the information in the record. Follow the agency's procedure if the patient requests to see the medical record. In many instances this is only available to the patient after discharge.

Basic Communication Review

A knowledge of the basic principles of therapeutic communication is essential for establishing rapport and trust, and to use specific techniques to facilitate interaction. Practice using therapeutic techniques whenever you can. Listen beyond the words and look for the feelings the patient is trying to convey.

Nonverbal Cues (What to Watch for). Watch for nonverbal communication in body posture, facial expression, gestures, hand movements, foot swinging, and so forth. Ask yourself if the nonverbal clues fit the words.

Verbal Cues (What to Listen for). Express interest and encouragement for what the patient is saying. Nod your head, maintain eye contact, and say "uh-huh" or "mmm." Lean slightly toward the patient. Use reflection for the feeling you sense behind the words and ask for feedback from the patient as to whether what you are perceiving is correct: "I sense that you are unsure about what to do." This allows the patient to validate or correct your impression.

Using Silence. Use silence appropriately; it gives the patient time to gather thoughts and formulate a response. Summarizing the highlights and main ideas of the interaction provides the patient with a chance to correct any misperceptions and to know clearly what has been relayed to the nurse.

Eliciting a Response. Use open-ended questions that will elicit more than a one- or two-word answer. Asking "who," "what," "where," or "how" requires the patient to elaborate when answering. Use "why" questions with caution, and rarely; they tend to make the patient feel defensive. Table 2-7 presents examples of therapeutic communication techniques and barriers to communication.

Helping the Patient Choose. Assist the patient to solve the problem. Do not give advice or opinions. Let the patient choose alternatives that appeal for solution of the problem. Help explore what those alternatives might be and then let the patient choose what is best. Table 2-8 provides some examples of therapeutic techniques.

First Contact: Approaching the Patient

Plan your first approach to the patient. If you are entering to take vital signs, be certain that you have all your equipment with you, including a piece of paper to write the results on. A "good morning, my name

TABLE 2-7 Quick Therapeutic Communication Review

Technique	Example	Rationale
Therapeutic Communication Techniques		
General leads	"Go on." "I see." "Uh-huh." "Please continue."	Encourages patient to continue or elaborate.
Open-ended questions or statements	"Tell me more about that feeling." "I'd like to hear more about...."	Encourages patient to elaborate rather than answer in one or two words.
Offering self	"I'm here to listen." "Can I help in some way?"	Shows caring, concern, and readiness to help.
Restatement	Patient says, "I tossed and turned last night." Nurse says, "You feel like you were awake all night?"	Restates in different words what the patient has said and encourages further communication on that topic.
Reflection	Patient says, "I'm so scared about the surgery; anesthesia terrifies me." Nurse says, "Anesthesia terrifies you?"	Reflecting same words back to patient. It also encourages further verbalization of feelings.
Seeking clarification	Patient says, "Seeing my little girl come visit me was so hard. I'm so upset." Nurse says, "Your daughter upset you?"	Seeks clarification if the little girl upset the patient or her leaving was the upsetting factor. Helps the patient clarify unclear thoughts or ideas.
Focusing	"Do you have any questions about your chemotherapy?"	Asking a goal-directed question helps the patient focus on key concerns.
Encouraging elaboration	"Tell me what that felt like." "I need more information about that." "Tell me more about the experience."	Helps the patient describe more fully the concern or problem under discussion.

Continued

TABLE 2-7 Quick Therapeutic Communication Review—cont'd

Technique	Example	Rationale
Giving information	"The test results take at least 48 hours to return to us." "You will get a preoperative injection that will make you sleepy before you are taken to the operating room."	Informs the patient of information relevant to specific health care or situation.
Looking at alternatives	"Have you thought about...?" "You might want to think about..." "Would this be an option?"	Helps patients see options and consider alternatives to make their own decisions about health care.
Silence	Patient says, "I don't know if I should have chemotherapy, radiation, or both." Nurse remains silent.	The nurse maintains silence, sitting attentively but quietly. This allows patients time to gather their thoughts and sort them out.
Summarizing	"You've identified your alternatives pretty clearly." "You are aware of the important signs and symptoms to report to your physician; plan to call to make an appointment next week."	Sums up the important points of an interaction.
Blocks to Effective Communication		
Changing the subject	Patient says, "I'm so worried about my husband." Nurse says, "It is time for your bath now."	Deprives the patient of the chance to verbalize concerns.
Giving false reassurance	"I'm sure it will turn out fine." "You don't need to worry."	Negates the patient's feelings and may give false hope, which, if things turn out differently, can destroy trust in the nurse.

Judgmental response	"I don't think that was a good thing for you to do considering you have diabetes."	Implies that the patient must take on the nurse's values and is demeaning to the patient.
Defensive response	Patient says, "My doctor never seems to know what is going on." Nurse says, "Dr. Smith is a very good doctor; he's here every day."	Nurse responds by defending the doctor. Prevents patients from feeling that they are free to express their feelings.
Asking probing questions	"Why were you there at that hour?" "What did you intend to prove?"	Pries into the patient's motives and therefore invades privacy.
Using clichés	"Cheer up, you'll be home soon." "This won't hurt for long." "You have a long life ahead of you."	Negates the patient's individual situation; stereotypes the patient. This type of response sounds flippant and prevents the building of trust between patient and nurse.
Giving advice	"If I were you, I would..." "I think you should..." "Why don't you..."	Tends to be controlling and diminishes patients' responsibility for taking charge of their own health.
Inattentive listening	Turning your back when the patient is sharing feelings or pertinent information; showing impatience with body language (i.e., tapping your foot or having your hand on the door to go out).	Indicates that the patient is not important; that the nurse is bored, or that what is being said does not matter.

Adapted from deWit S: *Fundamental concepts and skills for nursing*, ed 2, Philadelphia, 2005, Elsevier/Saunders, Chapter 7. Reprinted with permission.

TABLE 2-8 **Examples of Therapeutic Communication**

Patient	Nurse
	"How did it start?" "Tell me more about ..." (broad opening statements)
"I don't know what I'm going to do."	"You don't know what to do?" (reflecting) "Tell me what you have thought about doing." (exploring) "Let's look at your options."
(focusing)	
"I feel really rotten."	"Yes." "I see." "Uh-hmm."
(accepting)	
"That's what he said."	"Go on..." "Tell me more..." "Uh-huh..." (general leads)
"My whole family was here. My daughter finally came to see me. We got into an argument; it was silly. I couldn't sleep last night. I'm frightened."	"You couldn't sleep because of the argument?" "Being frightened kept you from sleeping?" (clarifying)
"I suppose this biopsy isn't anything to worry about. My sister's had several of them and they all were benign. I wish I could think about something else."	"You are worried about the biopsy and the possibility that the lump is not benign?" (verbalizing the implied)
"It will be so inconvenient for my family for me to go home while I still can't move around much. If I fall, they will feel guilty."	"You don't want to go home yet?" (focusing)
"I'll have to go through the chemotherapy and the radiation, but I'm sure not looking forward to it."	(Silence)

is _____ and I will be working with _____ (staff nurse) as your student nurse today" is one way to approach the patient. If it is the afternoon shift, just substitute "hello" for "good morning." Inquire how the patient slept last night or how the day has gone so far. Listen attentively. Express appropriate reactions or nod gently and then explain what you are going to do, and do it.

To interview the patient and gather the data you need for your assessment, explain that you have looked at the chart, but that your instructor requires that you ask a lot of questions that have probably already been asked by the physician or other nurses. Explain that it is part of your learning experience to interview patients yourself. When you have gathered the data you need, perform a beginning quick assessment following the guidelines in Table 2-9. This type of quick assessment should be

TABLE 2-9 Quick Head-to-Toe Assessment

At the beginning of each shift, each patient should be assessed quickly. This is often done along with the vital signs.

Initial Observation
Is the patient breathing?
Skin color
Appearance
Affect
How is the patient feeling?

Head
Level of consciousness
Appearance of eyes
Ability to communicate
Mentation status

Vital Signs
Temperature
Pulse rate; rhythm
Respiration rate, pattern, and depth
Oxygen saturation
Blood pressure; compare with previous readings

Pain Level per Use of Pain Scale; Location*
Abdomen
Shape
Soft or hard
Bowel sounds
Appetite
Last bowel movement
Voiding status

Extremities
Normal movement
Skin turgor and temperature
Peripheral pulses
Edema

Tubes and Equipment Present
Intravenous catheter: condition of site, fluid in progress, rate, additives
Oxygen cannula: liter flow rate
Pulse oximeter: intact probe; readings
Nasogastric tube: suction setting; amount and character of drainage
Urinary catheter: character and quantity of drainage
Dressings: location, drains in place, wound suction devices; character and amount of wound drainage
Traction: correct weight, body alignment, weights hanging free
Other equipment (CPM, SCDs, etc.)

Heart and Lung Assessment
Depending on time available and condition of patient, auscultation of heart and lungs may be done on initial assessment or later in the shift.

---

*Pain is assessed whenever vital signs are measured.
CPM, Continuous passive motion; *SCD*, sequential compression device.

done within the first hour of your shift. You will be able to gather further history and data about the patient as you interact with him or her throughout the shift. An in-depth physical assessment can be done a little bit at a time during the shift.

Assisting with the bath provides a prime opportunity to develop rapport with the patient and focus the conversation on his or her concerns. You can also do a good bit of physical assessment at that time—skin condition, range of motion of joints, ability to follow instructions, degree of alertness and cognition, and so forth. The main thing is to keep the interaction focused on the patient and not on yourself. There is a fine balance between the social interaction the patient needs and the professional interaction you need.

Learning from the Staff

The unit secretary or clerk can be an ally if you are kind and friendly to her or him; this is a person you want on your side. Address the person by name and be considerate. Don't interrupt her or his work if you can help it.

The charge nurse is ultimately responsible for the patients on the unit. This is the person to consult about patient assignments and problems. However, it is the staff nurse you will work with most closely. This nurse may be a registered nurse (RN) or an LPN/LVN. In either case, this person can teach you a lot. Remember that nurses have different personalities, strengths, and weaknesses just like everyone else. Some staff nurses like working with students more than others. Which type you have on any given day is not predetermined. If the staff nurse likes to teach, use her or his expertise to the maximum. If you are finished with your patient care, ask if you can shadow the staff nurse while he or she cares for other patients.

If you are working with a nurse who makes it obvious that a student is an inconvenience, just stay out of the way, keep the nurse posted on assessments and tasks completed for your patient, and use your instructor as your primary resource for the day. Sometimes people just may be having a bad day. Nurses may have a patient who isn't doing well, which might have them worried and preoccupied. It usually isn't a personal reaction toward you. Talk with your instructor about your feelings. Try to remember times when you have not wanted a younger sibling around or were angry with family members for one reason or another. Do follow the correct lines of communication, however; don't skip over this nurse with information that is needed about the patient. Remember to report off to the nurse at the end of the shift.

When other health care professionals come in to work with the patient, try to learn about what they are doing. Ask the respiratory therapist to show you more about the oxygen device in use. Watch the speech therapist work with the patient; then you can help the patient practice the exercises. Listen when the dietitian does diet counseling, and you will be able to reinforce the teaching with the patient. Go with the physician when he or she visits the patient. Stay out of the way and observe. Ask any questions after you have left the room.

Staying in the Good Graces of Your Instructor

Find out exactly what your instructor expects of you in the clinical area, and question any instructions you don't understand. Most instructors expect the following:

▼ Thorough preparation for the clinical experience
▼ Written work that is legible and neat
▼ A professional, clean, crisp appearance
▼ A friendly, quiet, professional demeanor
▼ Sufficient sleep before the clinical experience
▼ Promptness for clinical and conference
▼ Active participation in clinical conference
▼ A quick report on your patients when approached during the shift
▼ Cooperative team attitude with the staff
▼ Attentiveness to patient needs
▼ Appropriate, complete documentation
▼ Attentive listening and attention to instructions
▼ Seeking of skill experiences
▼ Taking responsibility for your own learning
▼ To find you in the patients' rooms when not charting, rather than sitting at the nurses' station
▼ You'll ask when you don't know how to do something, or whether it is permissible for you to do it
▼ To be notified immediately if something untoward happens or a mistake is made

If you happen to have an instructor that you can't seem to please, make an appointment and go talk about it. Ask what you can do to make the situation better. Tell her or him how you are feeling; your instructor is there to help you.

Preventing Errors and Harm to Patients

Always be attuned to patient safety factors. Keep side rails up when you are not at the bedside and the bed is raised. Remember to lower the bed when you have finished working with the patient. Always turn around when leaving the room and survey it. Does the patient have the call bell within reach? Are the items needed within reach?

Do not attempt to move an incapacitated patient by yourself unless you are certain that you can manage the correct technique for safe transfer. Get help—it isn't worth the risk of hurting the patient or yourself. You, in turn, can help others on the unit to move their patients. Learn to use the patient lifts that are available.

If you are told that a tube is to be removed from your patient, always check the chart **and read the actual order before taking the tube out.**

It is no fun having to reinsert a tube that is withdrawn in error, and it subjects the patient to unnecessary discomfort and risk of infection.

Follow the accepted "five rights–five responsibilities–three checks" method for administering medications. Perform the first two medication checks in the medication room or at the cart. Take the medication administration record (MAR) to the patient along with the medications and check the identification armband immediately on approaching the patient. Use an additional identifier (e.g., date of birth). Then check each medication appropriately with the MAR the third time just before giving it to the patient. Document that the medication has been given only after the patient has taken it.

Report abnormalities of vital signs immediately to the staff nurse assigned to the patient. Discuss anything else you find unusual or of concern about the patient. Talk with your instructor about your concerns also. It is better to have things checked out than to assume it is probably nothing to worry about.

Always report to the nurse when you leave the unit for a meal so that someone else will check on your patients while you are gone. Be certain your charting is caught up before you leave the floor.

Documentation Review

There are many different systems of documentation within clinical facilities today. You should receive information about the particular system used in your clinical facility and some guidelines for charting. If you don't, ask for this information. There should be a charting/documentation manual on the unit. Your documentation of patient care is a legal record; it needs to be legible, neat, and complete.

It is best to organize before beginning to write your nurse's notes. Chart from an outline format or chart from the data on your work organization sheet. Much information is recorded on flow sheets in the chart, such as the graphic record for vital signs, the intake and output (I&O) sheet, the daily activity or daily assessment form, the MAR, and so forth. However, in any documentation system, any abnormal findings must be recorded on the nurse's notes along with a description of what action was taken to correct the problem.

Most hospitals require that a nurse document data for each nursing diagnosis, problem, or "need" in the patient's chart at least once every 24 hours. For the nursing student, assessment data and actions should be recorded for each nursing diagnosis dealt with during that shift. General guidelines are listed in Table 2-10.

If the hospital or clinical site is using an electronic patient record system, find out how you are supposed to chart and what password to use to enter the system. Carefully read over what you have entered before pressing the "Enter" key or "OK." Log off the computer properly. **Never leave a computer without logging off.** Keep the computer screen out of the view of visitors in order to protect the patient's privacy.

TABLE 2-10 Documentation (Charting) Guidelines

Think of your charting as a camera that takes the patient's picture.

Organize Your Thoughts
▼ What have I seen that relates to this problem?
▼ What have I done about it?
▼ What do I plan to do about it? '
▼ How has my patient responded to what has been done?
▼ Do I have the right chart?

Build Your Planning on:
▼ Your initial assessment and further findings
▼ Your identification of the patient's problems
▼ Your patient care

General Guidelines
1. Chart neatly, legibly, and in blue or black ink.
2. Be brief, concise, accurate, and complete.
3. Use good grammar, correct spelling, correct punctuation, and proper terminology.
4. Note the time of each entry; also include month, day, year at the beginning of the shift charting.
5. Use a new line for each "new" (timed) entry. Put an ink line through extra space on the line you are charting on if you haven't used the entire line.
6. DO NOT ERASE. Draw a single line through an error; write "incorrect," "error," or "mistaken entry" over it; and sign your initials and the date (check agency procedure). Where there is room in the margin or above the corrected error, note the reason for it (i.e., "wrong chart," etc.).
7. When correcting or making a change to an entry in a computerized system, enter the current time and date, identify yourself, and note the reason for the change.
8. Never chart in advance of doing something; particularly do not chart medications before they are administered.
9. Include your signature and student designation (i.e., "S.N."). Use first initial and last name with that designation.
10. Leave out the word "patient." If the meaning of the entry is ambiguous, use the patient's name.
11. Use only those abbreviations accepted in your hospital (see the documentation manual).
12. Retain recopied pages in the back of the chart (i.e., corrected graphic record).
13. Check on the correct format for chart in your clinical facility.
14. Use flow sheets whenever possible—don't duplicate the information in the nurse's notes.
15. Use easily defined terms (e.g., "ate 75% of meal," rather than "ate well").
16. Rather than "tolerated well," state outcome: tolerated without pain, without nausea, or without complaint. ("Well" means different things to each of us.)
17. At the end of your shift, check through your charts and be certain that notes are complete, that entries on flow sheets are finished, and that each note is signed. Check through medication administration records (MARs) for your assigned patients and make certain that no medication has been overlooked and that you have initialed every medication you administered.

Continued

TABLE 2-10 Documentation (Charting) Guidelines—cont'd

Contents to Include

▼ Body care: type of bath, back care, skin care and assessment, mouth care, hair care, perineal care, position changes (most data go on flow sheets)

▼ Intake: diet, amount eaten, fluids (oral, nasogastric [NG], intravenous [IV]); IV site condition, type of fluid, equipment changed, complaints (use activity sheet, intake and output [I&O] sheet, IV flow sheet)

▼ Output: emesis, bowel movement, wound drainage, urine, vaginal flow, perspiration; include amounts and appearance (I&O sheet, nurse's notes)

▼ Treatments: time, type, duration, appearance of area treated, special equipment, specifics of procedures: how it is done, patient response; if left unit, time left, and by which conveyance; time returned

▼ Tests: laboratory specimens drawn; cultures, disposition of specimens, radiographs, sonograms, endoscopies, patient reaction, outcome if known, time left and returned to floor

▼ Dressings: appearance of incision or wound, smell, presence of drainage and appearance, how redressed and by whom

▼ Activity: time, ambulation and distance, exercises performed, including leg and breathing postoperatively, range of motion (ROM) performed, physical therapy, condition of pressure points, repositioning and for how long, and patient response to each

▼ Oxygen: time applied or amount changed, method of administration, safety precautions

▼ Medications: time, amount, route, response, any adverse reaction or side effects, ommision or delay, evidence of expected action (PRN and STAT doses are charted on the MAR, as well as the nurse's notes)

▼ Sleep: day or night; amount, interruptions; patient comments

▼ Mental state: mood, level of consciousness, general behavior (be objective)

▼ Preoperative preparation: teaching, physical preparation, time and by whom; patient questions

▼ Special conditions: traction, cast, special equipment—time applied, condition of patient, circulation checks and findings, skin condition, smell

▼ Vital signs: temperature, pulse, respiration, blood pressure; weight (on graphic record)

▼ Doctor's visits: examinations and treatments

▼ Visitors: who, how long, patient reaction

▼ Feelings: what patient states regarding feelings, complaints, concerns

▼ Physical assessment: what you see, hear, smell, and feel: auscultation of lungs, heart, bowel sounds, palpation of abdomen and pulses; inspection of skin, assessment of problem area in depth

▼ Safety factors: side rails up or down, replaced after working with patient; warnings; restraints in place

Giving a Report

When you leave your assigned unit for the day, you must report off to each nurse in charge of a patient assigned to you. If the nurse is on break when you are about to leave, report off to the charge nurse and make certain that it is understood you have not given report to the primary nurse for the patient. Table 2-11 provides an outline of the information you should supply to each primary nurse for your assigned patients.

DEVELOPING PROFESSIONALISM

Nursing is striving very hard to establish and maintain a professional image in the eyes of the public. The image you project as a nursing student, and then as a nurse, contributes to the overall public image of nursing. For this reason, nursing instructors will be teaching you about professionalism; they also will be evaluating you on your professional behavior.

There are three basic components of image: appearance, behavior, and verbalization.

Appearance

Appearance includes both clothes and grooming. Besides wearing the required uniform components, their cleanliness and neatness contribute

TABLE 2-11 Giving a Report

Organize your thoughts using an outline format before you give report to the staff nurse assigned to your patient.
State the following information:
▼ Patient name and room number
▼ Condition of patient (any changes) and last vital signs
▼ Diagnostic tests/surgery undergone
▼ Treatments or procedures done (including bath)
▼ As-needed (PRN) medications given and effect
▼ Intake and output (if ordered)
▼ Amount left to count in IV administration bag
▼ Appearance of IV sites
▼ Tubes in place and whether functioning properly; output
▼ Appearance of wounds and dressings in place; wound drainage output
▼ Bowel sounds present or absent
▼ Whether patient had a bowel movement
▼ Voiding status
▼ Any abnormalities of heart or lung sounds
▼ Pain/comfort status
▼ Any patient concerns
Be concise and professional.

IV, Intravenous.

to your image. Underwear should not be visible beneath a uniform, slips should not show beneath the skirt hem, buttons should not be missing, pocket corners should not be torn loose, hose should not have runs, shoes should be polished, shoelaces should be clean, and shoes should have quiet soles. Personal grooming of hair, beard, nails, and skin integrates with attire to project the visual image. The professionally groomed image includes keeping skin clean; wearing an effective, nonperfumed deodorant; and keeping nails clean and trimmed. Long nails make patients uneasy and are known to harbor bacteria. Infection control guidelines require that nail length be no more than one quarter inch. For men, the face should be clean shaven or the beard neatly trimmed. For women, wearing minimal, low-key makeup that projects a "business" look and refraining from working with chipped nail polish is important. Hair for both sexes should be secured so that it does not swing over the patient while performing care. Hair contains bacteria that can fall onto the patient. Jewelry also harbors microorganisms; only a plain wedding band should be worn in the clinical areas. Other types of rings and bracelets may injure the patient's skin while the nurse is giving direct care, and there is the chance of losing a stone or breaking a bracelet if it catches on something. A good guideline is not to wear any jewelry that dangles or can make noise. Perfumed lotions or colognes should not be used because they tend to cause nausea in people who are ill. Patients have a "clean and crisp" image of nurses, and they judge the nurse's competence by how the nurse looks and behaves.

Smoking. If a nursing student smokes at break, a breath freshener should be used before returning to the bedside; the smell of cigarettes to an ill nonsmoker is offensive. Cigarette smell also is carried on clothes back into patient areas. It is unprofessional to subject an ill person to this odor.

Dress. Student nurses are expected to dress professionally whenever they enter the clinical facility. This includes when students go to the units to obtain the data needed for their patient assignments. Although uniforms are not usually required when going to the hospital to gather patient data, a clean, pressed lab coat worn over professional clothes and a name tag are required. Jeans, shorts, miniskirts, T-shirts with slogans, sandals, spike high-heeled shoes, cowboy boots, and other such casual attire are inappropriate.

It is not considered professional to wear a nursing uniform when out with friends for a drink after the day's work is done. People do not know whether you have just finished a shift or are about to go on duty. A uniform worn while working in a clinical setting can be contaminated with many types of bacteria. It is best to change before running errands on the way home. The uniform truly should be worn only to and from clinical or work and while on duty.

Behavior

Behavior can add to your professional image or detract from it. Your facial expression, body language, and posture are components of your overall image. Chewing gum or eating while providing patient care is considered unprofessional. A cheerful smile, erect posture, and body language that indicates attentive listening and quiet efficiency instill a feeling of confidence in patients.

Preparation. Professional behavior also includes being well prepared for the clinical experience and turning in completed written work when it is due. Instructors expect students to come to the clinical experience on time, in correct attire, and with the tools of the trade—a working watch, a stethoscope, a pen, and bandage scissors.

Environmental Neatness. Attention to environmental care of the assigned patients' units and to the nurses' station and workrooms is another facet of professional behavior. Patient areas should be straightened at least once a shift. When time permits, add water to flowers to keep them fresh. Clean up after yourself in the medication room and at the nurses' station. Wipe up spills, throw away trash, and put equipment back where it belongs.

Attendance and Punctuality. Most nursing instructors consider the clinical experience equivalent to reporting to work. Absence is excused only for illness or a family emergency. It is not professional to miss clinical to study for an exam or take care of outside business matters. However, students are expected to remain at home if they are ill with something contagious such as a cold with fever, constant sneezing, coughing, or runny nose. Intestinal flu symptoms of vomiting or diarrhea should also signal the student to stay home. It is not professional to expose patients or colleagues to additional illness.

Cost Containment. Think cost-effectively. Return equipment no longer being used by patients quickly and see that charges for its use are stopped. Don't use a plastic medicine cup if a paper one will serve the same purpose. Check the patient's room for needed dressing or proce-dure supplies before taking new items from the clean supply area so that the least amount necessary is used. Continually ask yourself if there is a less expensive way to do the procedure. Remember to charge out supplies you use for the patient as required.

Verbalization

Appropriate verbalization is the third component of the professional image. Stress usually is high for the nursing student when in the clinical setting. It is necessary to make a conscious effort to stop and think before opening one's mouth when under such stress. Try to develop some quick stress relief techniques that you can use to calm yourself in particularly stressful situations. When with patients or staff, it is better to say too little than too much.

Patient Privacy. Remembering to provide privacy when interviewing a patient or performing a procedure builds trust between the patient and the nurse. Keeping the voice low when in the halls or at the nurses' station helps maintain the restful atmosphere the patients need.

Courtesy. Be courteous to other health care workers, as well as the patients. Saying, "may I," "please," "thank you," and refraining from directly interrupting another contributes to a professional image. Consideration of others is essential to professional behavior. You are there to meet the patient's needs, not to socialize. It is best to keep conversation and attention focused on the patient rather than on yourself or outside activities. Students should not clump together during clinical hours. Time is to be spent with the patients, studying the charts, or interacting with other health care professionals for the purpose of collaboration or learning.

Nonjudgmental Attitude. Another aspect of professionalism is development of a nonjudgmental attitude, be it toward patients or staff. Students sometimes find fault with nurses who do things differently than nursing school is teaching them. There are many right ways to perform different tasks. If the principles of asepsis and safety are followed, there is nothing wrong with performing a procedure in a different sequence or in a different way. Before loudly proclaiming that a nurse is doing something wrong, it is wise to discuss the matter quietly with the instructor.

Cultural Sensitivity. Patients and staff are not to be judged according to the student's values or cultural beliefs. Through the clinical learning process, students will become familiar with, and learn to respect, the values and beliefs of other cultures and individuals. In order to care for patients of different cultures, you must learn about the practices of cultural groups other than your own. By inquiring about cultural practices you observe, you can learn a great deal. There are many articles on practices within a variety of cultural groups. Several practical handbooks are also available. Assessment of cultural preferences should be a part of your nursing care. Never assume that just because a patient is part of an ethnic group that he or she adheres to that group's cultural practices. You must assess rather than assume.

Reporting Problems. It is professional to point out to the instructor if something has occurred with a patient that violates the principles of asepsis or safety. Current peer review criteria require that questionable practices or incidents be brought to the attention of the nurse involved and the supervisor. However, when in the student role, it is best to let the instructor handle such matters.

Honesty. Honesty is essential to professionalism. Students are encouraged to admit mistakes and be honest with everything that they do, including written work. It is unprofessional either to compose someone else's nursing care plans or other written assignments, or to have others contribute to yours. There are times when good students are encouraged to assist those having trouble with written work. Discuss the guidelines for this type of activity with the instructor before giving or getting assistance.

Professional behavior includes resisting passing along information on test questions to students in other class sections or allowing other students to copy from your answers. Such behavior is considered as much a form of cheating as copying answers from another student's exam paper.

Incorporating professionalism into one's behavior and nursing practice occurs over time. The student will benefit from observing the image, behavior, and verbalization of nurses who they perceive as being highly professional, and then attempting to model accordingly.

CLINICAL EVALUATION

Each nursing school has a form used to evaluate student performance in the clinical setting. Become familiar with this form during the first week of the semester. Also find the list of clinical objectives for the semester and review them each week to be sure you are meeting them.

Basic Competence

Initially, students are evaluated on their mastery of basic competence for particular skills. There often is a formal check-off evaluation period for various required skills done in the skills laboratory before the student ever attempts the skill in the clinical setting. Usually a skill is either passed or failed. If the student does not pass the skill check-off evaluation, remediation and practice are necessary before a second chance is given to pass the skill.

Once the student is caring for patients in a clinical setting, informal evaluation takes place on a weekly basis. This means that students are evaluated for competence and consistency of correct performance of skills previously evaluated in the skills lab or for adherence to principles taught in the lecture class (some schools do not have a skills laboratory). General concepts that are always undergoing constant evaluation, once they have been covered in theory class, include use of medical asepsis, communication, safety, legalities of practice, organization, and time management.

As content regarding various body systems is covered in theory class, the instructor will be evaluating your ability to apply the principles you have learned in the clinical setting. For example, once you have covered the basic concepts of disease and nursing care for the urinary system, you will be expected to be able to assist a patient to urinate, check for a full bladder, realize when a patient has gone too long without emptying the bladder, recognize signs that might indicate an infection, and determine when the color of the urine is abnormal. **Students sometimes fail to understand that they are going to be evaluated on synthesis and application of knowledge, as well as performance of skills.**

If you have difficulty in the clinical area and find that things seem not to be going right very often, immediately ask your instructor to meet with you and find out specifically what you can do to redirect the course of events. Admitting mistakes, taking positive steps to correct deficiencies, and being honest causes instructors to evaluate you more on *progress* than on individual instances in which things went wrong. In other words, you will be seen in a favorable light when you exhibit these behaviors.

Instructors often verbally tell students how they are doing every few weeks; if you do not get this type of feedback, ask for it. Try asking, "How am I doing? Is there any area in which you see that I need to improve to be at a passing level?" This will help you to relax more and stop worrying about what the instructor *might* be thinking.

Clinical Written Work

Written work is evaluated based on instructor expectations and course requirements. Items on the evaluation form usually indicate what will be evaluated on written work. For example, "Writes individualized nursing diagnoses pertinent to each patient's condition and problems" might be one item on the evaluation form. This would be appropriate for a first-semester student. Progress toward meeting this requirement would be shown by writing one or two correct nursing diagnoses on the first nursing care plan, writing two or three correct nursing diagnoses on the next care plan, and writing correct nursing diagnoses covering all of the patient's basic needs for the final care plan of the semester.

By the final course, the evaluation form might state, "Writes comprehensive nursing diagnoses in order of priority for assigned patients, considering psychosocial aspects of care, as well as physical condition and problems."

It is helpful to ask your instructor for a sample of the type and level of written work desired. This will provide you with an image of what is expected. Each nursing instructor has particular ideas about how the various parts of the nursing care plan should be done. Some instructors put more emphasis on one part than another. It is to your benefit to find out specifically what each instructor wants *before* you turn in your first assignment.

If there is a grading form to be used for the written work you are going to turn in, consult it to see that you have included everything that is required before completing the assignment. You don't want to lose points simply because you forgot to do a section of the assignment.

Formal Evaluation

A formal, summary type of evaluation usually is done at midterm and at the semester's end. At this time, the instructor will fill out the evaluation form and set a conference time to go over it with you. Often you will be asked to perform a similar self-evaluation. It is best to ask at the beginning of the semester if there will be a learning period and a specific evaluation period, so you will know what to expect. At formal evaluation time, you will be evaluated on your achievement of the objectives for the clinical experience, as well as for each item on the evaluation form. Usually there is a minimum level of competency expected from students at each level. This level is often defined by the course objectives. Instructors look for progress toward the course objectives, as well as for consistency in adherence to principles taught. If you do not feel that you understand the evaluation form, ask for a conference with your instructor during the first 2 weeks of school to clarify what is required of you.

Dealing with Stress

CONTROLLING STRESS

Becoming a nursing student automatically increases stress levels because of the complexity of the information to be learned and applied, and because of new constraints on time. There are several ways students can consciously decrease the stress associated with school. One way is to become very organized so that assignment deadlines or tests do not come as a sudden surprise. By following a consistent plan for studying and completing assignments, students can stay on top of requirements and thereby prevent added stress. Carry as few units as possible to lighten the study load.

Set Priorities

Another way to decrease stress while in school is to set personal priorities. Take time to survey all outside obligations and determine what can be given up during nursing school. Perhaps it would be best to concentrate solely on school if you are single and, if married or a parent, on school and family. That might mean restricting your social life or giving up many social activities such as being a Scout leader, Sunday school teacher, room mother at school, chief carpool driver, soccer coach, or Little League organizer. When school is completed, these extra roles could be taken up again. Adopt the motto *Keep It Simple* for your life while in school. The fewer outside distractions and responsibilities, the better your chances of success will be. Don't let housemates or dorm-mates constantly distract you.

Ask for Help

If you have family responsibilities, consider asking for assistance from family and friends during your school years. A lot of stress can be reduced if someone else will take over carpool duties for school-age children. Relatives and good friends may be willing to help with this task. A spouse may be able to help if work schedules permit. Relatives can act as representatives once in a while at a child's school function that falls on the eve of an important test. All household members can help with housekeeping, cooking, and errands. Adolescents can grocery shop from a list and children from the age of 9 years can prepare a simple dinner, even if it is hot dogs, scrambled eggs and biscuits, or TV dinners cooked in the microwave oven. Children can prepare their own school lunches, and could fix yours too! Things don't have to be perfect for these few years of school. Let go of ideals regarding meals and the state of living quarters or yard. The goal is to keep all occupants healthy and in touch with each other while you get through school. When a relative or dear friend asks what you would like for a special occasion gift, tell them you would like maid service to clean the house really well or a gardener to do some yardwork. Be creative with gift requests; ask for what you really need to decrease your stress.

Do One Task at a Time

Try to decrease your workload and maximize your time by handling items only once. Most of us spend a lot of time picking up things we put down rather than putting them away when we have them in hand. Going straight to the closet with your coat when you come in instead of throwing it on a chair saves you time in hanging it up later. Discarding junk mail immediately and filing the rest of your bills and such as they come in rather than creating an ever-growing stack saves time when you need to find something quickly. If all items requiring further attention are filed in some fashion, it helps you remember to take care of things on time rather than being so engrossed in your schoolwork that you forget about them. Many a nursing student has had the power, or the phone, cut off because the bill simply was forgotten.

Exercise

Regular exercise will also aid in stress reduction, even if it is only a 10-minute brisk walk each day. Where you may have been able to enjoy regular sessions at the health club or at an exercise class several times a week, you now may have to cut down on that time without giving up a set schedule for an exercise routine. Using an exercise bicycle that has a book rack on it at home, the YMCA, or a health club can help you accomplish two goals at once. You can exercise while beginning a reading assignment or while studying notes for an exam. Listening to lecture audiotapes while doing floor exercises is another option. At least a couple of times a week, however, the exercise routine should be done without the mental connection to school; time for the mind to unwind is necessary, too.

Stop for 10 Minutes

Taking 10 minutes a day away for yourself is very beneficial for stress reduction. Closing yourself in your room, lying down with eyes shut, and just free floating for a few minutes can revive energies and stop the whirlwind of thoughts of family obligations or nonstop tasks that tend to increase stress. Reading a few pages of a magazine or a book, listening to favorite music, napping for a short time, or doing a relaxation technique between the time you reach home and begin the evening routine can refresh both the body and the mind.

Prevent Preworry: Focus on Now

Another technique to help keep stress levels at a minimum is to stop worrying about things that cannot be changed. A great deal of energy is spent by many people on worrying about a situation that hasn't taken place yet. There will be time enough to worry about an event once it has actually occurred. Check yourself and see if you are a person who spends precious energy in this fashion. Wouldn't you rather spend that energy elsewhere? All of your preworry most likely will not change the event. Worrying about whether your teenager will have an accident while driving will not prevent such an event or cause it to happen. Worrying about whether a completed assignment will be graded favorably will not affect the grade. What is done is done. Try to focus on this day and this time, and do not worry about problems ahead of time. Deal with problems as they occur; if you cross that bridge before you need to, you will be paying the toll twice.

They Aren't Problems—They're Challenges!

Donald Tubesing, in his book *Kicking Your Stress Habits* (1981), talks about using the technique of relabeling to alter stress from bad to good. (This book is still in print and is available from Amazon.com.) He says that how you label experiences determines the effect of the experience on you. You have a choice as to how you view things. Labeling your clinical experience as exciting and challenging will make it far less stressful than labeling it as frightening and forbidding. If you label events as adverse during your daily crises, you end up with a batch of problems by the end of the day; if you label the same events as challenges, you end up with a bunch of opportunities. When something really seems stressful, ask yourself, "Will this matter in another 12 months? In 5 years?" This technique can quickly place things in a broader perspective.

Practice Self-Affirmation

A helpful method for decreasing test stress is to practice self-affirmation. After you have studied adequately and really do know the material, start looking in the mirror each time you pass one and say to yourself—preferably out loud—"I know this material and I will do well on the test." After several times of watching and hearing yourself reaffirm your knowledge, you gain inner confidence and are able to perform much better during the test period. This technique really works for students who are adventurous enough to use it. It may feel silly at first, but if it works, who cares?

Refuel and Recharge

The old standbys of enough sleep and adequate nutritional intake also help keep excessive stress at bay. Although nursing students learn about the body's energy needs in anatomy and physiology classes, somehow they tend to forget that glucose is necessary for brain cells to work.

Skipping breakfast or lunch or surviving on junk food puts the brain at a disadvantage. How can the student expect to grasp material when reading textbooks if the brain is operating in a glucose-deficient mode? Can a student perform in a top-notch manner in the clinical setting if the last meal was more than 8 hours ago? A car is not expected to run without gas; why should a body, and especially a brain, be expected to perform correctly when there is no fuel on board?

Once nursing classes start, students probably will not be able to obtain the same amount of sleep as they did before, but rest is essential to the body and brain for good performance. Think of it as recharging the battery. A run-down battery provides only substandard performance. For most students, it is better to spend 7 hours sleeping and 3 hours studying than to cut sleep to 6 hours and study for 4 hours. The improvement in the rested mind's efficiency will balance out the difference in the time spent studying. Knowing one's natural body rhythms is necessary when it comes to determining the amount of sleep needed for personal learning efficiency.

Know Your Internal Clock. Each student should determine if he or she is a "lark" or an "owl." Larks, day people, do best getting up early and studying during daylight hours. Owls, night people, are more alert after dark and can remain up late at night studying, catching needed sleep during daylight hours. It is better to work with natural biorhythms than to try to conform to an arbitrary schedule. You will absorb material more quickly and retain it better if you use your most alert periods of each day for study. Of course, it is necessary to work around class and clinical schedules. Owls should attempt to register in afternoon or evening lectures and clinical sections; larks do better with morning lectures and day clinical sections.

SPECIAL STRESSES
Danger of Infection

Becoming a nursing student brings special situations that many find very stressful. Patients do not always get well; sometimes they die, or lose body functions, which causes students considerable grief. Nurses care for patients with chronic or terminal diseases. Many diseases patients have can be contracted by the nurse. The disease most dreaded is acquired immunodeficiency syndrome (AIDS), caused by the human immunodeficiency virus (HIV). Working with AIDS patients and the potential for infection with HIV is very stressful for most health care workers. The following paragraphs present some information and suggestions for decreasing the fear of contracting harmful diseases and for dealing with dying patients.

Preventing Contraction of Disease. All health facilities have instituted the use of *standard precautions* to prevent health care workers from contracting harmful organisms through patient contact. The goal of standard precautions is to establish a barrier between the patient and anything that might transmit organisms to the worker or others. Personal protective devices such as latex gloves, masks, gowns, and goggles are used when exposure to body fluids that might contain HIV or hepatitis B or C virus is possible. Because it is not known which patients may harbor these harmful viruses, all patients are considered to be potential carriers, and standard precautions are used for every patient. Gloves are used when working with patients when there is any chance of coming into contact with blood, other body fluids, and secretions (except sweat). Students need to remember that dressings and linens may be contaminated, and gloves should be worn when handling these items. Table 3-1 presents standard precaution guidelines.

TABLE 3-1 Standard Precaution Guidelines

Human immunodeficiency virus (HIV), the virus that causes acquired immunodeficiency syndrome (AIDS), can be transmitted through exposure to infected blood or blood components and certain body fluids. Currently, there is no cure for AIDS and no immunization against it. The increasing prevalence of this disease increases the risk that health care workers will be exposed to blood from patients infected with HIV. The Centers for Disease Control and Prevention (CDC) recommends using *standard precautions*, formerly known as *standard blood and body fluid precautions*, for the care of all patients. These precautions are directed at preventing parenteral, mucous membrane, and nonintact skin exposures of health care workers to blood-borne pathogens such as HIV and hepatitis B virus (HBV). Because HBV causes serious illness (chronic hepatitis) and is known to predispose to cancer of the liver, immunization with HBV vaccine is recommended as an important adjunct to standard precautions for health care workers who may be exposed to blood. Other infection control measures are used in addition to standard precautions. The following is a summary of the CDC guidelines.

Body Fluids to Which Standard Precautions Apply
Standard precautions apply to blood; semen; vaginal secretions; and cerebrospinal, synovial, pleural, peritoneal, pericardial, and amniotic fluid and tissues. Blood is the single most important source of HIV, HBV, and other blood-borne pathogens in the health care facility. Standard precautions also apply to feces, nasal secretions, sputum, tears, urine, and vomitus. General infection control measures apply to the handling of these body fluids. Sweat is the only body fluid to which standard precautions do not apply. Proper handwashing is mandatory.

General Precautions
1. Use standard precautions for all patients.
2. Use appropriate barrier precautions routinely when contact with blood or other body fluids of any patient is anticipated.

Continued

TABLE **3-1 Standard Precaution Guidelines—cont'd**

▼ Wear gloves when touching blood and body fluids, mucous membranes, or nonintact skin; when handling items or surfaces soiled with blood or body fluids; and when performing skin sticks such as injections, finger or heel sticks, venipuncture, and other vascular access procedures.
▼ Change gloves after contact with each patient.
▼ Do not reuse gloves.
▼ Do not wash or disinfect surgical or examination gloves for reuse.
▼ Wear masks and protective eyewear or face shields during procedures that are likely to generate drops of blood or other body fluids to prevent exposure of mucous membranes of the mouth, nose, and eyes.
▼ Wear impermeable gowns or aprons during procedures that are likely to generate splashes of blood or other body fluids.
3. Take precautions to prevent injuries caused by needles, scalpels, and other sharp instruments or devices during procedures; when cleaning used instruments; when disposing of used needles; and when handling sharp instruments after procedures.
    ▼ Discard needle units uncapped and unbroken after use.
    ▼ Place disposable syringes and needles, scalpel blades, and other sharp items in puncture-resistant containers.
    ▼ Place puncture-resistant containers as close as practical to areas of sharp use.
4. Even though saliva has not been implicated in the transmission of HIV infection, a barrier should be used for mouth-to-mouth resuscitation, or a resuscitation bag should be used. Mouthpiece barriers, resuscitation bags, or both should be available for use in areas in which the need for frequent resuscitation is probable, such as the emergency department.
5. If exudative lesions of the skin or weeping dermatitis is present, refrain from all direct patient care and from handling patient care equipment without gloves until the condition resolves.

Handwashing
Handwashing is the hallmark of preventing the spread of infectious organisms. The CDC has recently modified the handwashing guidelines.
▼ Wash hands after touching blood, body fluids, secretions, excretions, and contaminated items, whether or not gloves are worn.
▼ Wash hands immediately after removing gloves.
▼ Wash hands between patient contacts and when otherwise indicated to avoid transfer of microorganisms to other patients or environments.
▼ Wash hands after handling potentially contaminated items.
▼ It may be necessary to wash hands between tasks and procedures on the same patient to prevent cross-contamination of different body sites.
▼ Use a plain (non-antimicrobial) soap for routine handwashing.
▼ Use an antimicrobial agent or a waterless antiseptic agent for specific circumstances (e.g., control of outbreaks or hyperendemic infections), as defined by the infection control program.

Precautions for Invasive Procedures
▼ Use appropriate barrier methods—gloves, surgical mask, protective eyewear, face shield, gown, and apron—when participating in invasive procedures.

TABLE 3-1 Standard Precaution Guidelines—cont'd

▼ Wear disposable, impervious shoe coverings when there is massive blood contamination on floors, and wear gloves to remove the coverings.

▼ When performing or assisting at a delivery, wear gloves and a gown when handling the placenta or the infant until blood and amniotic fluid have been removed from the infant's skin, and use gloves during postdelivery care of the umbilical cord.

▼ If a needlestick occurs through a glove or a glove becomes torn, remove it and don a new glove as quickly as patient safety permits.

Environmental Considerations

▼ Standard sterilization and disinfection procedures currently recommended for use in health care settings are adequate.

▼ Sterilize instruments or devices that enter sterile tissue or the vascular system before reuse.

▼ Clean and remove soiled areas on walls, floors, and other surfaces routinely; extraordinary attempts to disinfect or sterilize are not necessary.

▼ Use chemical germicides approved as hospital disinfectants (and tuberculocidals) to decontaminate spills of blood and other body fluids. In the absence of a commercial germicide, a solution of sodium hypochlorite (household bleach) in a 1:10 dilution is effective.

Precautions with Soiled Linens

▼ Handle soiled linen as little as possible and with minimum agitation to prevent gross microbial contamination of the air and of persons handling the linen.

▼ Place linen soiled with blood or body fluids in leak-resistant biohazard bags at the location at which it was used.

Handling Specimens

▼ Place all specimens of blood and listed body fluids in well-constructed containers with secure lids to prevent leakage during transport.

▼ Be careful not to contaminate the outside of the container when collecting specimens.

Infective Waste Disposal

▼ Incinerate or autoclave infective waste before disposal in a sanitary landfill.

▼ Carefully pour bulk blood, suctioned fluids, excretions, and secretions down a drain connected to a sanitary sewer.

Data from U.S. Department of Health and Human Services, Public Health Service, 1989. Update: Garner JS: *Hospital Infection Control Practices Advisory Committee: guideline for isolation precautions in hospitals,* Atlanta, 1996, Public Health Service, U.S. Department of Health and Human Services, Centers for Disease Control and Prevention. Modified April 1, 2005.

Basic Self-Protection. Self-protection against all disease is provided by following all infection control guidelines within the clinical facility. *Good hand hygiene* is the most effective method of reducing transfer of microorganisms from one person or object to another. Getting into the habit of washing hands after each patient contact, before gloving, and when gloves are removed is one way to help decrease fear of contracting harmful organisms.

Working with AIDS Patients. Developing an understanding of HIV and how it is transmitted is primary for decreasing the stress of working with an AIDS patient. Standard precautions are all that are necessary when having direct patient contact. The student should focus on the AIDS patient as a person with needs just like any other patient. Remembering to think through a procedure carefully before beginning it will help the student use proper barrier precautions, such as gloves, goggles, mask, and gown, when needed. Whenever working with needles or other sharp objects, the student should remember to move slowly and carefully to prevent sticks. When working with a known HIV-positive individual and blood contact is probable, it is best to use a double-gloving technique if gloves are vinyl, or to use high-quality latex gloves. Never assume that blood will not splash inadvertently into your eyes or mouth, touching your mucous membranes. It is better to wear goggles and a mask than to be directly exposed to the virus.

Keeping the immune system in top functioning order should be a priority for all nursing students and nurses. This is accomplished by getting sufficient sleep, eating properly balanced meals, exercising regularly, attending to minor illnesses quickly, and keeping stress levels within limits. Along with the use of standard precautions, boosting the immune system is the best protection against HIV.

As for the stress of working with all the problems that AIDS patients often have, the student must study the disease and the multiple system problems it causes. Skillful care, good assessment, and therapeutic communication are essential components of providing the AIDS patient with compassionate, comprehensive nursing care.

Working with Dying Patients

First experiences with patients who are dying are very stressful for most students. Prepare yourself by knowing what you can do to help the patient. Be familiar with the stages of grief and dying, while realizing that each patient deals with impending death very individually. Primarily, the nurse's role is to provide basic care and comfort for the patient. Attend to small tasks such as lubricating lips, straightening linen, offering a back rub or a foot rub, straightening the environment, making certain enough warmth is provided, and offering sips of fluid, for example. Provide adequate pain relief. Check with the patient about what he or she desires.

Psychologically, the nurse assists the patient through the stages of the coping process, helping the patient face issues as honestly as possible by being supportive. All you need to do in this area is let the patient know that you are available to talk about whatever is pertinent. Never force a subject on the patient. Be honest and ask questions cautiously about what the patient knows and feels. Take cues from the patient about what topics are acceptable to explore. Do not avoid the issues of the illness, complications, or impending death. The patient may need someone to talk with about these things who is not personally involved.

Sometimes it is helpful to reminisce with the patient, going through his or her life and remembering the major landmarks and fun times. Encourage family members or significant others to do this with the patient as well. Best of all, just offer yourself by simply being there for the patient. Check his or her needs often and offer just to sit quietly in the room as time permits.

Discuss any fears you have with your instructor. Be specific about questioning what to do in certain situations. Know what to expect with a particular patient as death approaches. Will breathing become labored? Will the skin become mottled? Will the patient become unconscious? Ask the nurse caring for the patient about the probable course for this patient. Knowing what to expect can greatly decrease your fear of the actual event. Also clarify your role in the event that the patient stops breathing or has a cardiac arrest. Usually you should stay with the patient and use the call system to call out for the primary nurse or charge nurse. Always determine whether the patient has a do-not-resuscitate (DNR) order. If such an order has not been written, you must begin cardiopulmonary resuscitation as soon as a respiratory or cardiac arrest is observed, even though it is known that the patient is terminally ill.

Special Patient Situations

Being prepared to deal with patients who are depressed, hostile, aggressive, or manipulative can also help decrease stress on clinical days. Your nursing texts tell you how to determine if a patient is depressed or manipulative, but you will probably be able to pick out hostile and aggressive patient behaviors from your own life experience.

Depressed Patients. Nursing interventions that sometimes help depressed patients include the following:
▼ Sit with the patient quietly.
▼ Encourage performance of activities of daily living; assist as needed.
▼ Work slowly; be patient and gentle.
▼ Point out the patient's strengths and accomplishments; emphasize good qualities.
▼ Do not admonish the patient to "cheer up and look at the bright side of things"; don't be overly bright and cheerful.
▼ Encourage social interaction, particularly exercise.
▼ Be alert for signs of self-destruction and the potential for suicide.

Manipulative Patients. Manipulative patients use a variety of means to get what they want from the nurse. This behavior has various causes. It may be the way the patient has learned to communicate or respond to stress; often, the patient simply fears losing control. Some specific nursing interventions useful in dealing with the manipulative patient include the following:

▼ Respond to the inappropriate behavior as calmly as possible; set limits. If the patient is shouting, explain that the shouting is inappropriate, is disturbing to other patients, and makes it impossible to help. Say, "Please stop shouting and tell me how I can help you."

▼ Be consistent and firm. State *how often* you can check on him or her; restate this as needed when a demand is made between scheduled times.

▼ Do not become defensive; do your best not to take insults personally. Establish a personal emotional distance, but not professional distance.

▼ Be aware of how this behavior affects you. The patient may remind you of previous experiences with manipulative family members or friends.

▼ When all else fails or if you get into a shouting match that will promote further hostility, tell the patient you are leaving the room because of his or her behavior and that you will be back when he or she has calmed down. State when you will be back and then arrive on time.

Hostile Patients. Hostile, aggressive behavior includes verbal or physical threats. This type of behavior is usually an attempt to maintain control over the situation. When another person becomes aggressive, the usual response is to become defensive. Aggressive behavior occurs in family members as well as patients at times. Some helpful nursing interventions to use when these behaviors occur include the following:

▼ Let the person know you are aware of his or her anger; allow feelings to be expressed freely. Ask what is upsetting the person and inquire what can be done to help him or her feel less angry and frustrated. *Actively* listen. Do not place blame.

▼ Provide opportunity for the patient to make suggestions about self-care; give in to demands that are not unreasonable.

▼ Encourage as much physical activity as possible to help release pent-up feelings.

▼ Allow the patient to make decisions and choices regarding his or her care or the timing of procedures and tasks of daily living. This provides a sense of power and control.

▼ Rather than responding to the content of what the person is ranting about, attempt to respond to the underlying feelings.

▼ When a patient raises his or her voice, lower yours. Treat the person as an adult.

▼ Do not make promises that cannot be kept. This destroys trust. Protect your safety if a situation escalates by taking the following actions:

▼ Maintain a safe distance from the patient while verbally interacting (at least an arm and a half's length away); maintain eye contact.

▼ Position yourself between the patient and the exit; keep your hands in sight.

▼ Remove potential weapons from the patient's reach; remove your stethoscope from around your neck.

Working with the Patient Who Has Difficulty Communicating Verbally

You may find it stressful to be assigned to care for a patient who is aphasic and has difficulty communicating owing to brain injury from a stroke or head trauma. There are several different varieties of aphasia (expressive, receptive, global, mixed), and patients experience the problem from a slight to a profound degree. Your nursing texts can give you specific suggestions for dealing with individual types of aphasia, but here are some general guidelines:

▼ Keep the environment as relaxed and quiet as possible.
▼ Assume the patient can understand what is heard even though speech is jargon (nonsensical) or the patient is mute.
▼ Speak to the patient on an adult level; do not treat the patient as mentally incompetent.
▼ Talk to the patient, not about the patient to someone else in the room.
▼ Face the patient, establish eye contact, and speak slowly and distinctly without dropping your voice level at the end of sentences; do not shout.
▼ Give short, simple directions; use pantomime and body language to enhance the words.
▼ Phrase questions so that they can be answered with a yes or no, and look for nonverbal behavior that agrees with the patient's answer.
▼ Give the person time to respond to questions; processing may be slower than usual.
▼ Do not ask more than one question at a time.
▼ If there is a need to repeat something, use the same words the second time. If there is still difficulty, phrase what was said differently.
▼ Use body language to enhance your message.
▼ Allow one person to speak at a time.
▼ Be very patient.

Remember that the person may get very frustrated when he or she is unable to verbalize adequately. A statement such as, "It must be very difficult and frustrating not to be able to make people understand what you want to say," and a caring touch may help. Remembering what it must be like for the person may help keep you from becoming short and impatient. Be aware that aphasia worsens with anxiety or fatigue.

Personal Safety to and from Work and School

Nurses often work shift hours and must travel in the dark. General safety rules for driving and walking should be followed.

▼ Keep car doors locked at all times.
▼ Look in the backseat before entering the car.

▼ Have the car door key out and ready before you depart from the building.

▼ Be certain to keep the gas tank at least one-quarter full at all times; keep the car in good running condition.

▼ Travel on well-lighted, busy streets, avoiding isolated back roads or troubled parts of town.

▼ If you are being followed, drive to the nearest open business for help, or drive to the police or fire station.

▼ Park only in areas that are well lighted; when leaving the clinical facility, walk with several other people or ask the security guard to accompany you during early morning or nighttime hours.

▼ Do not stop to aid a stranger in a stalled vehicle; proceed to an open business and report the stalled vehicle to the police.

▼ If you have vehicle trouble, raise the hood, get back in your vehicle, and lock it. Turn on the flasher. When someone offers assistance, roll down the window only enough to talk and ask the person to call a relative, friend, garage, or the police for you. Never get into a stranger's car.

When Walking

▼ Avoid walking alone; don't keep looking down, walk with your head up, shoulders back, and survey your surroundings; make eye contact with passers-by.

▼ Stay in well-lighted, pedestrian-traveled areas; avoid shortcuts through alleys, parks, vacant lots, or deserted areas.

▼ If someone stops and asks for directions, maintain distance, and especially do not approach a stopped car.

▼ If you are being followed, briskly walk to the nearest business or residence for help.

▼ If you are bothered by people in a car, turn and walk the other way.

▼ Women should hold a purse close and securely; avoid carrying extra money or valuables on your person.

▼ Have your door key ready before leaving your car to enter your home.

▼ Be alert; note the people around you, your surroundings, and the total environment.

Rape Prevention and Response. Classes in personal defense are offered at most colleges and in many communities. A few hours spent learning methods of defense can prevent injury or rape. Following the preceding safety tips when walking and driving also can help prevent rape. However, should you be threatened with rape, there are some things that may prevent its occurrence. Active resistance is one way, and it must be used very quickly. The purpose is to startle or surprise your attacker. For active resistance, use whatever you have as a weapon. Kick, scream, yell, or run; use your keys, purse, or whatever you have. A spray device with mace, tear gas, or pepper is effective, and nurses or students who have to walk to distant parking lots would be wise to have such a device in hand before leaving the building. Most such devices will attach to your key ring.

Should rape occur, call the police *immediately*. Also call the local rape crisis center for quick counseling and a support person. It is important to *not* take a bath or shower. Physical evidence, including seminal fluid, hairs, scrapings of flesh from under fingernails, and any of the attacker's blood on the victim, is necessary for positive identification of the attacker and a court conviction. The police will ask for information about the car the attacker was driving, including make, color, and license plate number; the attacker's race, approximate age, weight, height, color and length of hair, and color of eyes; clothing worn, including hat, tie, shirt, pants, shoes, and glasses; and any unusual marks, scars, tattoos, or rings. Knowing whether the attacker is right-handed or left-handed is also helpful.

SELF-ASSESSMENT
Assessing Your Stress Level

Sometimes no matter what stress reduction techniques are used, the stresses of keeping up with classes, clinical, family, and job can become too much. Keep a finger on the pulse of your stress by assessing your stress status about once a month. Ask yourself the following questions:

▼ Are you easily angered by uncontrollable events such as being put on hold on the phone, traffic jams, persistent poor weather patterns, or malfunctioning equipment?

▼ Do you feel rushed all the time because tasks seem never to end?

▼ Has your sleep pattern changed? Do you have difficulty falling or staying asleep?

▼ Has your eating pattern changed? Have you lost or gained weight?

▼ Are you tired, anxious, or feeling burned out all the time?

▼ Do you suffer from chronic headaches, backaches, stiff neck or shoulder, or intestinal or stomach complaints?

▼ Do you often find yourself clenching or grinding your teeth?

▼ Are you drinking or smoking more than usual?

▼ Do you often lose your temper or burst into tears without a really good reason?

▼ Are you constantly irritable?

Addressing Your Stress

If the answer is yes to three or more of these questions, sit down and really evaluate how you can decrease the stress levels in your life. If you don't think you can change anything, seek professional assistance. Your school has counseling available from instructors and school counselors. You pay for these services when you register for your classes, so use them. Don't wait to go for help; the quicker you resolve the problem, the better your chance for success in school.

Using a relaxation technique will help you keep stress levels under control. However, the technique must be used regularly several times a week until it becomes second nature for it to be useful (Tables 3-2 and 3-3).

TABLE 3-2 Guided Imagery for Relaxation

This is a sample script for a guided imagery experience. It can be recorded on audiotape and replayed while doing the exercise. Writing your own script and recording it maximizes the experience. When recording your script, read slowly in a soft but audible voice. Pause sufficiently after each instruction and section to allow time for following the instruction or forming the mental image. Performing this guided imagery exercise regularly can reduce stress.

When performing the exercise, sit or lie down and stretch out. Reduce noise and other distractions as much as possible. Dimming the light in the room is beneficial.

Script

▼ Close your eyes and gently relax.
▼ Take a deep, slow breath. Feel your lungs fill with clean, fresh air. Slowly exhale, sending all tension out with the air you exhale.
▼ Take another deep, slow breath; let it out slowly, sending body tension with it.
▼ Visualize yourself walking on a path in the woods at the edge of a meadow.
▼ Smell the clean air, the forest, the flowers in the meadow.
▼ Feel the warmth of the sun and the soft, warm breeze. Hear the crunch of pine needles under your feet. It is so peaceful and serene here.
▼ You approach a brook, gently gurgling over the rocks in its path. You listen to the pleasant sound of the running water. It is almost as if the brook talks to you, welcoming you to this beautiful place of peace, comfort, and serenity.
▼ You look at the grass and moss growing in beautiful greens beneath the water.
▼ Patches of sunlight filtering through the trees warm your body. What a perfect spot to enjoy.
▼ You find a comfortable place, spread the blanket you were carrying, and sit and gaze at the trees, the meadow, the blue sky with fluffy white clouds slowly moving to the horizon. What a beautiful place.
▼ You listen to the birds calling to each other and contemplate their cheerful melodies.
▼ A butterfly flits across your field of vision. You watch it as it zigzags across the meadow, going from flower to flower.
▼ It is so warm, pleasant, and peaceful here. You remember other days in similar surroundings.
▼ You concentrate on the feelings of warmth and peace the sun and breeze convey to you. Happiness fills your heart and soul and you realize you can return here anytime you wish. This place is yours.
▼ Replenished, you arise, fold the blanket, and prepare to return up the path.
▼ You look around you once more—at the trees, the meadow, the sky, the brook—imprinting the scene in your memory to take with you. This is your special place; it will always be here for you.
▼ You walk slowly up the path through the sunlight toward home.
▼ When you are ready, open your eyes.

TABLE 3-3 Relaxation Exercise

This exercise is performed by recording the script onto audiotape and following the instructions as the tape is played. Using the exercise regularly over a period of weeks makes it easier to call on these techniques to induce relaxation during an exam or at other times you feel particularly tense.

Slowly read the script in a soft, firm voice. Allow sufficient pauses between segments for the instructions to be followed. Sit in a chair or lie down to do the exercise. Decrease outside noise and distractions as much as possible.

Script

▼ Close your eyes and find something to focus on mentally. It might be a spot of light, your pulse, a visual image, or whatever you choose. Try to hold it constant.

▼ Breathe in slowly and deeply; hold it a moment, and slowly breathe out. Now breathe normally, slowly, in and out.

▼ Tighten your face and neck muscles as firmly as you can, while clenching your teeth. Feel the tension. Hold it; slowly relax the muscles. Feel the relaxation in your face, jaw, and neck.

▼ With less tension, tighten the muscles in the face, jaw, and neck again. Feel this level of tension. Let go and relax. Notice the feeling of relaxation.

▼ Tighten your chest muscles firmly. Hold it; feel the tension. Let the chest muscles relax. Notice the difference between the tension and relaxation.

▼ Tighten the chest muscles again with less tension. Now let the muscles relax. Feel the relaxation.

▼ Tighten the fists and arm muscles as hard as possible. Hold the tension a moment. Slowly relax the muscles. Notice the difference in feeling between tension and relaxation.

▼ Tighten the fists and arm muscles again with less tension. Hold it. Let the muscles relax. Feel the relaxation.

▼ Tighten the abdominal muscles firmly. Hold the tension, noting the feeling. Relax the muscles, noting the difference between tension and relaxation.

▼ Tighten the abdominal muscles again with less tension. Hold it. Allow the muscles to relax completely. Notice the feeling of relaxation.

▼ Tighten the muscles in your right leg and foot. Hold the tension. Note the feeling. Allow the muscles to relax. Notice the difference between tension and relaxation.

▼ Tighten the muscles in your right leg and foot again with less tension. Hold it. Completely let go of the tension in the muscles and relax. Feel the relaxation.

▼ Tighten the muscles in your left leg and foot firmly. Hold it. Note the tension. Allow the muscles to relax. Focus on the difference between tension and relaxation.

▼ Tighten the muscles in your left leg and foot again with less tension. Hold it. Completely let go of the tension in the muscles and relax. Notice the feeling of relaxation.

▼ Breathe in and out deeply and slowly five times, focusing on your breathing.

▼ When you are ready, open your eyes.

Continuing Your Education

TAKING THE NEXT STEP
Types of Programs

Many colleges offer a ladder program within the nursing division. Some begin with a certified nursing assistant (CNA) curriculum that progresses to a 1-year practical nurse program. When that is completed, the student has the option to complete a second year for an associate degree or continue for a bachelor's degree in nursing (BSN).

A number of colleges and universities offer a BSN completion program for associate degree nursing (ADN) graduates. These programs generally take 1 to $1\frac{1}{2}$ years to complete the nursing part of the curriculum. Sometimes the completion program can be accomplished via distance learning. Excelsior College (formerly Regent's College of New York) and Jacksonville University both offer distance learning programs. The Web site at http://distancelearn.excelsior.edu lists many colleges with distance learning courses in nursing. The College Network is another place where many types of nursing programs are available for completion via distance learning. The Web site at www.college-net.com lists the various options under "Nursing."

Traditional BSN programs require 4 to 5 years for completion. These usually provide a more rounded education with required courses in the arts, as well as the sciences. The nursing courses usually do not begin until after the first 2 years of study. Students who are already licensed nurses may receive credit for some previous nursing courses.

Returning Students

Returning to school is a big step. If you have been out in the workforce for many years, the student role will be a bigger adjustment for you than for those who recently graduated from a nursing program. The written work required for an associate degree registered nurse (AD RN), BSN, or BSN completion program is extensive, and there is a heavy emphasis on the nursing process. You will review the nursing process during the first few weeks of class. Do your best to develop an even better understanding of each component, how it works, and how the five parts are integrated with the application of the whole circular process. Spending time now to review the nursing process, especially as it relates to paperwork, will save you considerable time and frustration throughout your nursing classes and clinical courses.

Differences in Training

There will be an even greater emphasis on the development and use of critical thinking throughout your nursing courses. If you graduated many years ago and have been out working as a licensed nurse, it would be wise to read about critical thinking skills. Most fundamentals of nursing texts address this content. There are several very good books on the market aimed particularly at critical thinking in nursing. *Critical Thinking and Clinical Judgment: A Practical Approach*, third edition (2004), by Rosalinda Alfaro-LeFevre is one.

The RN student is expected to learn in-depth assessment skills. Emphasis will be placed on extensive history taking and skillful, thorough, physical assessment. Compared with the licensed practical nurse/licensed vocational nurse (LPN/LVN), the RN is expected to develop even greater expertise in identifying problems and detecting complications and changes in patients' condition. If it has been some time since you used all of your physical assessment techniques, practicing them on friends and relatives is the best way to brush up on and improve your skills.

The BSN student studies more in-depth supervisory and management content than the AD RN student. The BSN also is trained in community health and research techniques. A course in statistics is usually required. Some BSN curricula require more science and math courses as well.

Differences in Curriculum and Demands

Your ADN or BSN curriculum will be similar to the previous nursing curriculum, but it will be more comprehensive. The volume of reading is time consuming, and there is much written work to be completed. Try to cut your work schedule to 20 hours a week or less. Aim for success from the beginning. If you have spare time after part-time work, and you see that your class average is good, you can slowly increase your work hours. Only rarely can students with family commitments be successful in an RN program while working full time. Many single students who do not have other obligations have difficulty keeping up with school if they try to work 40 hours per week. Students who are single parents often need to work more hours, but they are at a disadvantage because they are the only caregiver for the family. This seriously limits available study time. Relatives sometimes can be asked to take total charge of the children for several hours, thereby providing blocks of study time one or more times a week for the months you are in school.

What You Bring with You: Skills and Habits

Depending on where you have been working, you will have some advantages over the brand new nursing students. If you have been working in a hospital or long-term care facility, you should be confident and competent with skills such as administering medications, catheterization, nasogastric tube insertion, and so on. You should also have an advantage in that you are familiar with many prescription drugs.

Sometimes instructors prefer that a skill be performed differently than you learned it years ago. Protocols and ideas on the best way to do things change from time to time as new information emerges. If you learned a procedure differently in your previous nursing courses, you may have to practice outside of class time to learn to perform the skill in a new way.

If you have been working in home care and using your assessment skills regularly, you may have an advantage over other students in this area. You function independently and make decisions, and you have developed good people skills and know how to adapt to various situations.

The student who has been working in long-term care is very familiar with the problems and needs of the elderly and with ways of efficiently caring for this population. For example, you know the techniques that are helpful in administering medications to the person who has a decreased ability to swallow, how to distract the patient who has decided not to do what you want him or her to do, and how to quickly clean up the bed and skin of an incontinent patient.

The nurse who has years of experience in the operating room is very comfortable and confident with sterile technique. You have an idea of why the patient has postoperative pain and why joints and muscles are sore and stiff after lengthy surgery. You are familiar with the routine of assisting with a cardiac or respiratory arrest.

Catching up with Generic Students

Unless you work in an area in which you deal with a large variety of drugs, you will need to spend extra time refreshing your pharmacology knowledge when you enter an ADN or BSN program. The generic students have had many months to study drugs. You should start refreshing your memory about a set number of drugs each week from the first week. Learn the drugs first by classification. If you understand how the class of drugs works, you can determine the possible side effects and then determine the probable nursing implications. After you have learned the classification information, choose individual drugs that differ in side effects or nursing implications from the general drugs of the class, and learn those.

One problem many returning students have is adopting the student role when they are in clinical. Each student should clarify with the instructor which skills can be done without supervision and which skills the instructor must be called on to observe. It is so natural to perform a procedure while working as a licensed nurse that, as a student, it is easy to forget you can't just go and do it. Get into the "think before doing" mode during your clinical experience hours.

Role Transformation

As you near the end of the RN curriculum, you will be learning more advanced supervision of others. Advanced leadership skills are part of the RN competencies. Sometimes it is difficult for a practical nurse who has little supervisory experience to act in a leadership role. One way to prepare for leadership is to observe continually how the charge nurse and staff RNs interact and delegate tasks to the other personnel on the unit. Role play for yourself how you would handle various situations and assignments within your daily work routine. Observe the nuances of supervision in action.

The BSN student should begin to see the larger picture from the standpoint of administration and the institution. This requires a broadened mind-set. As an AD RN, the focus is on providing patient care. As a BSN, the focus expands to include the needs of the nursing unit and the institution, as well as the patient. Aspects of the new role will include learning to schedule personnel, managing conflicts among staff, writing policies, and performing evaluations of staff. There will be more emphasis on long-term quality improvement.

Try to mainstream yourself with all the students rather than segregating yourself with other returning practical nurses or ADN nurses. In this way you can glean anything that the other students learned during their courses that you received credit for because of your previous nursing courses. You can find out which instructors might suit your needs and personality best, and you will have some assistance in refining your paperwork from those who already have been through some of it. Share your expertise when asked; it will boost your morale. You have a lot to offer to the learning experience of the group.

Consistently using the *Student Nurse Planner* for scheduling your time for study and other activities can help you achieve success in the nursing program, whether you are a returning practical nurse, an AD RN, or a beginning BSN nursing student. Success begins with planning.

Aids to Success

COMMUNICATION AND WORD LISTS
Prefixes and Suffixes Used in Medical Terms

Term	Meaning	Term	Meaning
Combining Form		**Prefixes**	
adeno-	gland	a-, an-	without, away from, not, no
alveolo-	air sac	ab-	away from, absent
andro-	man, male	ana-	up, back, again
angio-	vessel	ante-	before
appendic/o	appendix	auto-	self
arthro-	joint	bi-	two, twice
audio-	hearing	co-, con-	with, together
bio-	life	contra-	opposite, against
broncho-	bronchus	dia-	through, complete
carcino-	cancerous	dys-	difficult, painful, abnormal
cardio-	heart	ec-, ecto-	outside, out
ceco-	cecum	endo-, ento-	within
cephalo-	head	epi-	above
cerebro-	brain	exo-	out
cervico-	neck	hyper-	excessive, above
chole-	bile	hypo-	below, deficient
cholecysto-	gallbladder	meta-	change, over, after
claviculo-	clavicle	peri-	around, surrounding, about
colo-	colon	pro-	before, in front of
cranio-	skull	re-	back, again
cutaneo-	skin	retro-	behind, backward
cysto-	bladder, sac	sym-, syn-	together, with
dermato-	skin	trans-	across, through, beyond
duodeno-	duodenum		
encephalo-	brain	**Suffixes**	
entero-	intestine	-ac	pertaining to
erythro-	red	-al	pertaining to
esophago-	esophagus	-algia	painful condition, pain
gastro-	stomach	-cele	hernia, swelling, sac
gingivo-	gums	-centesis	puncture of a cavity
gluco-	sugar	-cyte	cell
gyneco-	woman	-desis	fusion, binding, fixation
hemato-	blood	-ectasis	expansion, dilation

Continued

Prefixes and Suffixes Used in Medical Terms—cont'd

Term	Meaning	Term	Meaning
Combining Form—cont'd		**Suffixes—cont'd**	
hepato-	liver	-ectomy	excision, removal of a body part
hystero-	uterus		
laryngo-	larynx	-emia	blood
leuko-	white	-genic	origin, formation
lipo-	fat	-gram	the record made, mark
meningo-	membrane	-graph	instrument for recording, machine
myelo-	marrow, spinal cord		
		-graphy	the process, process of recording
myo-	muscle		
naso-	nose	-ia	condition
nephro-	kidney	-iasis	morbid condition
neuro-	nerve	-ic	pertaining to
onco-	mass, tumor	-ist	one who specializes in
oophoro-	ovary	-itis	inflammation
ophthalmo-	eye	-logy	process of study
orchio-	testis	-lysis	dissolution, setting free
osteo-	bone	-malacia	softening, soft
oto-	ear	-megaly	enlargement
patho-	disease	-oid	form, shape
pharyngo-	pharynx	-ology	study or science of
pneumo-	lung, air	-oma	tumor
procto-	rectum, anus	-opsy	viewing
prostato-	prostate	-osis	condition, disease
psycho-	mind	-pathy	disease, suffering
pyelo-	kidney	-penia	deficiency, lack of, decrease
radi-	ray, radiation		
rhino-	nose	-pexy	fixation
salpingo-	tube	-plasty	mold, shape, repair
spleno-	spleen	-ptosis	downward displacement, falling
stoma-	mouth		
thrombo-	clot	-rhea	flow, discharge
thyro-	thyroid	-scope	instrument to visually examine
tracheo-	trachea		
tricho-	hair	-scopy	process of examining
uretero-	ureter	-sis	state of, condition
uro-	urine	-spasm	involuntary spasm
vertebro-	vertebra	-stasis	control, constant level
		-stomy	creation of an opening
		-therapy	treatment
		-tome	instrument for cutting
		-tomy	process of cutting
		-trophy	nourishment

Adapted from Anderson DM, Keith J, Novak PD, Elliot MA, editors: *Dictionary of medicine, nursing and health professions*, ed 7, St Louis, 2006, Mosby. Reprinted with permission.

Commonly Used Abbreviations

Abbreviations

ad lib—as desired
ADLs—activities of daily living
AMA—against medical advice
amb—ambulate
ax—axillary
BP—blood pressure
C—centigrade
c/o—complains of
dx—diagnosis
ETOH—alcohol
F—Fahrenheit
h—hour
HOB—head of bed
HOH—hard of hearing

H&P—history and physical
Hx—history
I&O—intake and output
IV—intravenous
LLE—left lower extremity
LUE—left upper extremity
NG—nasogastric
NV—nausea and vomiting
OOB—out of bed
OT—occupational therapy
P—pulse
PT—physical therapy
q—every
R—respirations

RLE—right lower extremity
ROM—range of motion
RUE—right upper extremity
SS—social service
T—temperature
TCDB—turn, cough, and deep breathe
TED—thromboembolic disease
tx—treatment
VS—vital signs
wt—weight
×—times

Symbols

∆—change
↑—increase, up

↓—decrease, down
⊕—positive, present

⊖—negative, not present

Medication Routes

IM—intramuscular
IV—intravenous

PO—by mouth
PR—by rectum

subcut—subcutaneous

Medication Frequency

AC—before meals
bid—twice a day

PC—after meals
PRN—as needed

qid—four times a day
tid—three times a day

Medications

ASA—aspirin
NSAIDs—nonsteroidal antiinflammatory drugs

Medication Dosages

g—gram
gr—grain
gtts—drops

L—liter
mEq—milliequivalent
mg—milligram

mL—milliliter
tsp—teaspoon

Serum Laboratory Tests

CBC—complete blood count
C&S—culture and sensitivity
ESR—erythrocyte sedimentation rate

Hct—hematocrit
Hgb—hemoglobin
K^+—potassium
Na—sodium
PT—prothrombin time

PTT—partial thromboplastin time
RBCs—red blood cells
WBCs—white blood cells

Other Terms

AO×3—alert, oriented to person, place, date, and time
c—with

C—cervical
CSF—cerebrospinal fluid
HA—headache
L—lumbar

MVA—moving vehicle accident
s—without
STAT—immediately

Continued

Commonly Used Abbreviations—cont'd

Diseases

ALS—amyotrophic lateral sclerosis
Ca—cancer
CP—cerebral palsy

CVA—cerebrovascular accident
MS—multiple sclerosis
TIA—transient ischemic attack

Diagnostoic Tests

CAT or CT—computerized
  axial tomography or
  computed tomography
EEG—electroencephalogram

EMG—electromyography
MRI—magnetic resonance imaging
PET—positive emission tomography

Adapted from Anderson DM, Keith J, Novak PD, Elliot MA, editors: *Dictionary of medicine, nursing and health professions*, ed 7, St Louis, 2006, Mosby. Reprinted with permission.

Basic Spanish Phrases

Do you speak English?
¿Habla Usted inglés?
ah-blah oo-stehd een-glehs?

I don't understand.
No entiendo.
noh ehn-t-yehn-doh.

My name is …
Me llamo …
meh yah-moh …

Speak more slowly, please.
Hable mas despacio, por favor.
ah-bleh mahs dehspahs-yoh, pohr fah-vohr.

Do you understand?
¿Entiende Usted?
ehn-t-yehn-deh oo-stehd?

Are you allergic to anything?
¿Es usted alérgico(a) a cualquier cosa?
ehs oo-stehd ah-alehr-hee-koh(kah) ah kwahl-k yehr koh-sah?

Do you take any medications?
¿Toma medicamentos?
toh-mah meh-dee-kah-mehn-tohs?

Here is the call light.
Aquí está la luz para llamar a la enfermera.
ah-kee eh-stah lah looss pah-rah yah-mahr ah lah ehn-fehr-meh-rah.

This is the television control.
Este es el control de la televisión.
ehs-teh ehs ehl kohn-trohl deh lah teh-leh-vee-s-yohn.

Basic Spanish Phrases—cont'd

This is the bed control.
Este es el control de la cama.
ehs-teh ehs ehl kohn-trohl deh lah kah-mah.

Don't get out of bed by yourself.
No se baje de la cama solo (a).
noh seh bah-heh deh lah kah-mah soh-loh (ah).

You may not eat or drink anything more before surgery.
No comerá o beberá nada antes de la cirugia.
noh koh-meh-rah oh beh-beh-rah nah-dah ahn-tehs deh lah
    see-oo-hee-ah.

Do you have pain?
¿Tiene dolor?
t-yeh-neh doh-lohr?

Are you nauseated?
¿Siente el estómago revuelto?
s-yehn-teh ehl ehs-toh-mah-goh reh-vwehl-toh?

Take a deep breath in, please. Exhale.
Respire profundo, por favor. Exhale.
reh-spee-reh proh-foon-doh, pohr fah-vohr. ehks-ah-leh.

Now cough.
Ahora tosa.
ah-or-a toh-sah.

I am going to give you an injection.
Le voy a poner una inyección.
leh voy ah poh-nehr oo-nah een-yehk-s-yohn.

I have some medications for you to take.
Tengo unas medicinas para que Usted las tome.
tehn-goh oo-nahs meh-dee-see-nahs pah-rah keh oo-stehd lahs toh-meh.

When was your last bowel movement?
¿Cuándo tuvo su último excremento?
kwahn-doh too-vah soo ool-tee-moh ehks-kreh-mehn-toh?

I need to measure your urine.
Debo medir su orina.
day-bow meh-deer soo oh-ree-nah.

It is time for your bath.
Es hora de su baño.
ehs oh-rah deh soo bahn-yoh.

Continued

Basic Spanish Phrases—cont'd

Do not pull on the tube.
No jale el tubo.
noh hah-leh el too-boh.

Sit up, please.
Siéntese, por favor.
s-yehn-teh-seh, pohr fav-vohr.

NURSING CARE AND DOCUMENTATION
Application of the Nursing Process

The five-step nursing process (Figure 5-1) is set in motion at the time of the initial assessment. There is continuous interaction among the components. The patient is the center and focus of all activities within the process. Arrows point in both directions, indicating that the process is always in motion. Thus each component is subject to revision as new information is obtained through interaction with the patient.

From deWit S: *Fundamental concepts and skills for nursing,* ed 2, Philadelphia, 2005, Elsevier. Reprinted with permission.

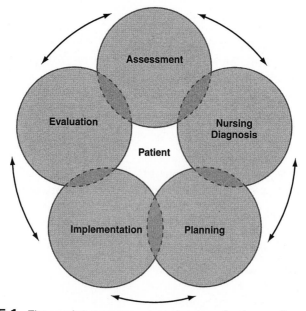

FIGURE 5-1 The nursing process—an overlapping, circular, continuous process centering on the patient.

Application of the Nursing Process—cont'd

Examples of Activities for the Five Steps of the Nursing Process

Assessment
Data gathering
  Initial admission assessment
  Interview and history taking
  Physical examination/assessment
  Measure vital signs
  Chart review
Beginning of shift, quick head-to-toe assessment
Focused assessment for major problem (e.g., respiratory, cardiac)
Assessment of equipment needed for a procedure
Assessment of learning needs
Review of literature
  Review of anatomy and physiology of body systems involved in client
    problem
  Read about disease process or surgery
  Consult other health team members for further information

Nursing Diagnosis
Analysis of data to determine problem areas
Definition of problems
Formulation of nursing diagnoses (RN)
Recognition of appropriate nursing diagnoses chosen for care plan
  (LPN/LVN)
Collaboration with client for prioritization of problems/nursing diagnoses

Planning
Write goals/expected outcomes for each nursing diagnosis
Set a time for expected outcomes to be met
Plan interventions to assist client to meet expected outcomes or achieve goals
Devise a teaching plan
Check physician's orders to see what needs to be done
Plan ahead for surgical care
Plan ahead for medication administration
    Check to see that medications are on the unit
    Verify medication orders on the medication administration record (MAR)
      with the physician's original orders
Collaborate with other health team members to plan client's total care
  for the shift
Document the nursing care plan
Plan revision of interventions when evaluation indicates the need
Plan work organization for the shift

Intervention (Doing)
Supervise implementation of the nursing care plan
Carry out planned nursing interventions
Delegate tasks to ancillary nursing personnel
Perform skills and procedures
    Measure and record intake and output (I&O)
    Change a dressing

Continued

Application of the Nursing Process—cont'd

Examples of Activities for the Five Steps of the Nursing Process—cont'd

Intervention (Doing)—cont'd
Apply a heat treatment
Give medications
Teach clients
Counsel assigned clients and families
Consult/collaborate with other health team members (e.g., social worker, dietitian, pharmacist, physician)

Evaluation
Evaluate client condition
Evaluate effect of nursing interventions
Determine if nursing interventions are assisting client to meet expected outcomes/goals
Evaluate whether interventions need to be revised
Evaluate effect of treatments
Evaluate data to see if there is progress toward recovery
Evaluate for side effects and therapeutic effect of medications
Document evaluation data
Evaluate whether work organization schedule needs to be revised

NANDA Nursing Diagnoses 2007-2008

Activity intolerance
Activity intolerance, Risk for
Airway clearance, Ineffective
Allergy response, Latex
Allergy response, Risk for latex
Anxiety
Anxiety, Death
Aspiration, Risk for
Attachment, Risk for impaired parent/infant/child
Autonomic dysreflexia
Autonomic dysreflexia, Risk for
Body image, Disturbed
Body temperature, Risk for imbalanced
Bowel incontinence
Breastfeeding, Effective
Breastfeeding, Ineffective
Breastfeeding, Interrupted
Breathing pattern, Ineffective
Cardiac output, Decreased
Caregiver role strain
Caregiver role strain, Risk for
Comfort, Readiness for enhanced
Communication, Impaired verbal

NANDA Nursing Diagnoses 2007-2008—cont'd

Communication, Readiness for enhanced
Conflict, Decisional
Conflict, Parental role
Confusion, Acute
Confusion, Chronic
Confusion, Risk for Acute
Constipation
Constipation, Perceived
Constipation, Risk for
Contamination
Contamination, Risk for
Coping, Compromised family
Coping, Defensive
Coping, Disabled family
Coping, Ineffective
Coping, Ineffective community
Coping, Readiness for enhanced
Coping, Readiness for enhanced community
Coping, Readiness for enhanced family
Decision making, Readiness for enhanced
Denial, Ineffective
Dentition, Impaired
Development, Risk for delayed
Diarrhea
Dignity, Risk for Compromised Human
Disuse syndrome, Risk for
Diversional activity, Deficient
Energy field, Disturbed
Environmental interpretation syndrome, Impaired
Failure to thrive, Adult
Falls, Risk for
Family processes: Alcoholism, Dysfunctional
Family processes, Interrupted
Family processes, Readiness for enhanced
Fatigue
Fear
Fluid balance, Readiness for enhanced
Fluid volume, Deficient
Fluid volume, Excess
Fluid volume, Risk for deficient
Fluid volume, Risk for imbalanced
Gas exchange, Impaired
Glucose level, Risk for unstable
Grieving
Grieving, Complicated

NANDA Nursing Diagnoses 2007-2008—cont'd

Grieving, Risk for Complicated
Growth, Risk for disproportionate
Growth and development, Delayed
Health behavior, Risk Prone
Health maintenance, Ineffective
Health-seeking behaviors
Home maintenance, Impaired
Hope, Readiness for enhanced
Hopelessness
Hyperthermia
Hypothermia
Identity, Disturbed personal
Immunization status, Readiness for enhanced
Incontinence, Functional urinary
Incontinence, Overflow urinary
Incontinence, Reflex urinary
Incontinence, Stress urinary
Incontinence, Total urinary
Incontinence, Urge urinary
Incontinence, Risk for urge urinary
Infant behavior, Disorganized
Infant behavior, Readiness for enhanced organized
Infant behavior, Risk for disorganized
Infant feeding pattern, Ineffective
Infection, Risk for
Injury, Risk for
Injury, Risk for perioperative-positioning
Insomnia
Intracranial adaptive capacity, Decreased
Knowledge, Deficient
Knowledge, Readiness for enhanced
Lifestyle, Sedentary
Liver function, Risk for impaired
Loneliness, Risk for
Memory, Impaired
Mobility, Impaired bed
Mobility, Impaired physical
Mobility, Impaired wheelchair
Moral distress
Nausea
Neglect, Unilateral
Noncompliance
Nutrition, Readiness for enhanced
Nutrition: less than body requirements, Imbalanced

NANDA Nursing Diagnoses 2007-2008—cont'd

Nutrition: more than body requirements, Imbalanced
Nutrition: more than body requirements, Risk for imbalanced
Oral mucous membrane, Impaired
Pain, Acute
Pain, Chronic
Parenting, Impaired
Parenting, Readiness for enhanced
Parenting, Risk for impaired
Peripheral neurovascular dysfunction, Risk for
Poisoning, Risk for
Poisoning, Risk for perioperative
Post-trauma syndrome
Post-trauma syndrome, Risk for
Power, Readiness for enhanced
Powerlessness
Powerlessness, Risk for
Protection, Ineffective
Rape-trauma syndrome
Rape-trauma syndrome, compound reaction
Rape-trauma syndrome, silent reaction
Religiosity, Impaired
Religiosity, Readiness for enhanced
Religiosity, Risk for impaired
Relocation stress syndrome
Relocation stress syndrome, Risk for
Role performance, Ineffective
Self-care, Readiness for enhanced
Self-care deficit, Bathing/hygiene
Self-care deficit, Dressing/grooming
Self-care deficit, Feeding
Self-care deficit, Toileting
Self-concept, Readiness for enhanced
Self-esteem, Chronic low
Self-esteem, Situational low
Self-esteem, Risk for situational low
Self-mutilation
Self-mutilation, Risk for
Sensory perception, Disturbed
Sexual dysfunction
Sexuality pattern, Ineffective
Skin integrity, Impaired
Skin integrity, Risk for impaired
Sleep, Readiness for enhanced
Sleep deprivation

NANDA Nursing Diagnoses 2007-2008—cont'd

Social interaction, Impaired
Social isolation
Sorrow, Chronic
Spiritual distress
Spiritual distress, Risk for
Spiritual well-being, Readiness for enhanced
Stress overload
Sudden Infant Death Syndrome, Risk for
Suffocation, Risk for
Suicide, Risk for
Surgical recovery, Delayed
Swallowing, Impaired
Therapeutic regimen management, Effective
Therapeutic regimen management, Ineffective
Therapeutic regimen management, Ineffective community
Therapeutic regimen management, Ineffective family
Therapeutic regimen management, Readiness for enhanced
Thermoregulation, Ineffective
Thought processes, Disturbed
Tissue integrity, Impaired
Tissue perfusion, Ineffective
Transfer ability, Impaired
Trauma, Risk for
Urinary elimination, Impaired
Urinary elimination, Readiness for enhanced
Urinary retention
Ventilation, Impaired spontaneous
Ventilatory weaning response, Dysfunctional
Violence, Risk for other-directed
Violence, Risk for self-directed
Walking, Impaired
Wandering

Determination of Erikson's Stages of Development

Nursing students are often asked to place the patient within one of Erikson's stages of development by listing some behaviors to verify the correct stage. The following chart provides a listing of sample behaviors that are appropriate for each stage.

Determination of Erikson's Stages of Development—cont'd

Trust vs. Mistrust

Trust
Verbal behaviors
"I believe you."
"I know I can tell you ..."
"You will help me."
"You are my friend."

Nonverbal behaviors
Asking for help with the expectation of receiving it. Accepting help from others comfortably. Sharing time, opinions, emotions, and experiences.

Mistrust
Verbal behaviors
"I am afraid of you."
"I can't tell you about anything."
"You cheat."

Nonverbal behaviors
Inability to accept help. Confining conversation to superficialities. Rigidly controlling behavior so that only that which is socially approved is exhibited. Refusal to share time, experiences, opinions, and emotions.

Autonomy vs. Shame and Doubt

Autonomy
Verbal behaviors
"I will."
"I won't."
"Okay, I'll do it myself."
"This is my opinion."
"I can wait."

Nonverbal behaviors
Tries to dress self or perform other tasks on own. Accepting group rules but able to express dissent when it is felt. Accepting leadership role when it is appropriate. Expressing own opinion. Accepting postponement of wish gratification easily. Ability to cooperate. Demonstrates some self-control.

Shame and Doubt
Verbal behaviors
"My opinion doesn't count."
"I never know the answers."
"I don't want to hear what you have to say."
"I must be right."
"I should do that."

Nonverbal behaviors
Overly concerned with being clean. Not maintaining own opinion when opposed. Failing to express needs. Maintaining own opinion despite adequate proof to the contrary. Lacks self-control. Unable to wait; hoarding; soiling. Being vindictive.

Initiative vs. Guilt

Initiative
Verbal behaviors
"Let me try."
"What is it; how does it work?"
"Where does that road go?"
"May I wash my hair?"

Nonverbal behaviors
Exploring. Starting new projects with eagerness. Expressing curiosity. Being original. Ability to evaluate own behavior. Brushes teeth without being told.

Guilt
Verbal behaviors
"I'm afraid to do that."
"You go first and I will follow."
"I'm ashamed to make a mistake."

Nonverbal behaviors
Imitating others rather than developing ideas independently. Expressing a great deal of embarrassment over a small mistake. Always taking the blame.

Continued

Determination of Erikson's Stages of Development—cont'd

Industry vs. Inferiority

Industry

Verbal behaviors

"I'm working on this. When it is done I will start on that."
"I like to be busy."
"Group projects are fun."
"I'm going to do my homework now."

Nonverbal behaviors

Completing a task once it is started. Working well with others. Using time effectively. Feelings of competence. Good self-esteem.

Inferiority

Verbal behaviors

"I can't work with other people."
"I have a lot of things going but nothing finished."
"I don't think I can do it."

Nonverbal behaviors

Not completing any set tasks. Not contributing to the work of the group. Not organizing work. Avoids responsibility.

Identity vs. Role Diffusion

Identity

Verbal behaviors

"I'm going to be a nurse."
"I believe in these principles."
"I think mothers should do this and fathers should do that."
"I know where I'm going."
"I feel good about myself."

Nonverbal behaviors

Establishing relationships with the same sex and then with the opposite sex. Planning realistically for the future. Reexamining values. Asserting independence. Trying various things.

Role Diffusion

Verbal behaviors

"I don't know who I am."
"Where am I going?"
"Is it better to be male or female?"
"I don't know what I mean."

Nonverbal behaviors

Failing to differentiate roles or goals in life. Failing to assume responsibility for directing own behavior. Imitating others indiscriminately. Accepting the values of others without question.

Intimacy vs. Isolation

Intimacy

Verbal behaviors

"We are very close friends."
"I love Dan."
"My family is very close."
"I have lots of good friends."

Nonverbal behaviors

Establishing a close and intense relationship with another person. Acting out and accepting appropriate sexual behavior as desirable. Maintaining a marital or other monogamous relationship.

Isolation

Verbal behaviors

"I'm a loner."
"I don't need anyone."
"I don't care about anyone."
"I'm very lonely."

Nonverbal behaviors

Remaining alone. Not seeking out others for companionship or help. Avoiding sex role by remaining nondescript in mannerisms and dress.

Determination of Erikson's Stages of Development—cont'd

Generativity vs. Stagnation

Generativity

Verbal behaviors	*Nonverbal behaviors*
"John and I have agreed to have two children."	Productive. Maintaining employment. Parenting. Accepting interdependence.
"He has his work and I have mine ... together we make a team."	Guiding others. Creative. Community or church leadership. Completes creative endeavors; has hobbies.
"I am raising three children."	Performs own self-care and takes
"I am employed at ..."	responsibility for own health.
"I love to sew."	

Stagnation

Verbal behaviors	*Nonverbal behaviors*
"I can't hold a job."	Not listening to others because of need
"I don't want to learn about it."	to talk about oneself. Constantly losing
"I haven't time to volunteer."	employment. Showing concern only
"You do it; I'm going out."	for oneself despite the needs of others.
"That's too bad, but it isn't my problem."	Self-absorption. Always finds excuses. Refuses to learn self-care.

Integrity vs. Despair

Integrity

Verbal behaviors	*Nonverbal behaviors*
"Life has been very good to me."	Using past experiences to guide others.
"I can't do the things I once did, but I enjoy other things."	Accepting new ideas. Accepting limitations. Maintaining productivity in some area. Exploring philosophy
"I enjoy discussing current events."	of living and dying. Enjoying some aspect of things as they are.
"I read the newspaper every day."	Actively participating in own care as much as able.
"I love watching the birds at the feeder."	
"I enjoy seeing my children and my grandchildren."	

Despair

Verbal behaviors	*Nonverbal behaviors*
"I am no use to anyone."	Crying; being apathetic and listless.
"Everyone is gone—my family, my friends."	Not developing any new interests beyond a few routine activities.
"What is the use of living; I can't do anything."	Developing no new relationships. Not accepting changes. Limiting
"Everything I did is gone now. Why did this happen?"	interpersonal contacts. Demanding unnecessary help and attention.
"These new ways are no good."	Remaining in pajamas and robe all the time.

Descriptive Terms Used in Nurse's Charting

Word	Idea to Be Charted	Terms Suggested
Abdomen	Appearance	Distended, round, flat, soft, firm, hard, rigid, protruding, flaccid, tympanic, distended, tender, boardlike, bruised, or ecchymotic (terms are interchangeable)
Bleeding	In very large amounts or spurts	Spurting blood, profuse oozing
	Very little	Minimal amount
	Location	Blood in vomitus (hematemesis), blood in urine (hematuria), blood in sputum, nosebleed, or epistaxis
Breath	Taking air in	Inspiration
	Breathing air out	Expiration, exhalation
	Short time without breathing	Apnea
	Rapid breathing	Hyperpnea
	Cannot breathe lying down	Orthopnea
	Snoring sounds of breathing	Stertorous respiration
	Unpleasant odor	Halitosis
	Increasing dyspnea with periods of nonbreathing	Cheyne-Stokes respiration
	Difficulty breathing or labored breathing	Dyspnea
Convulsion	Muscles contract and relax	Clonic tremor or convulsion
	Muscle contraction maintained for a time	Tonic tremor or convulsion
	Localized muscle contraction	Spasm
	Began without warning	Sudden onset
	Abrupt start and end of spasm or convulsive seizure	Paroxysm
Cough	Various types of coughing	Tight, loose, deep, dry, hacking, painful, exhaustive, hollow
	Coughs all the time	Continuous
	Coughs over long period of time	Persistent
	Coughs up material	Productive
	Coughs without producing material	Nonproductive
	Sudden attacks of coughing	Paroxysmal
Conscious-ness	Aware of surroundings	Alert—conversant, fully awake and conscious
	Partly conscious	Groggy, lethargic, semiconscious
	Arousable but not conscious; responds to some stimuli	Stuporous, semiconscious; responsive to verbal stimuli, responsive to tactile stimuli

Descriptive Terms Used in Nurse's Charting—cont'd

Word	Idea to Be Charted	Terms Suggested
	Unconscious, cannot be aroused; does not respond to stimuli	Comatose
Drainage	Water, from the nose	Coryza
	Sticky	Viscous
	Bloody	Sanguineous
	Contains serum and blood	Serosanguineous
	Fecal (contains bowel material)	Fecal
	Contains mucus and pus	Mucopurulent
	From vagina after delivery	Lochia
Odor	Not pleasant; pungent; spicy like fruit	Aromatic Fruity
	Unpleasant	Offensive; foul
	Smelling like a particular thing	Characteristic of …
Pain	Amount of pain	Use statement of patient; slight to severe; rate on a scale of 1 to 10
	Types of pain	Aching, dull, slight, burning, throbbing, gnawing, acute, chronic, generalized, superficial, excruciating, unyielding, cramping, darting, colicky, continuous, shifting, agonizing, piercing, intense, cutting, transient, localized, remittent, persistent
	Comes in seizures	Spasmodic
	Spreads to certain areas	Radiating
	Begins suddenly	Sudden onset
	Hurts when moving	Increased by movement
Skin	Terms to describe condition	Pale, pink, red, moist, dry, clear, coarse, tanned, scaly, thick, loose, rough, tight, infected, discolored, jaundiced, mottled, calloused, edematous, excoriated, abraded, bruised, painful, scarred, black, oily, brown, white, clammy, rash, wrinkled, smooth
Speech	Unable to be understood	Incoherent
	Meaningless	Rambling, irrelevant
	Runs words together	Slurs
	Difficulty in speaking	Dysphasia
	Unable to speak	Aphasia
	Other terms to describe	Stammering, stuttering, hoarse, feeble, fluent, clear

Guidelines for Discharge Teaching

Cover the following points when performing discharge teaching:
▼ Care of incision if present
▼ Dressing changes; supplies; techniques; soiled dressing disposal
▼ Care of tubes, drain suction devices, other equipment in place
▼ Care of IV site
▼ Activity level permitted; restrictions
▼ When can return to work
▼ Driving restrictions
▼ Sexual activity guidelines
▼ Weight lifting restrictions
▼ Bathing/showering—precautions
▼ Rest requirements
▼ Diet guidelines; any restrictions
▼ Signs and symptoms to report
▼ When and where to make follow-up appointment
▼ Medications, purpose, schedule, side effects to report
▼ Where to obtain medical equipment to be rented or purchased
▼ Number to call if questions arise

Writing a Discharge Summary

Follow your agency's format and guidelines regarding content. The following points are usually included in the discharge summary, which is written in the nurse's notes or on a discharge sheet:
▼ A summary of the patient's care
▼ An outline of all patient teaching, including what the patient was taught about diagnosis, diet, activity, medications, wound care, special care, signs and symptoms of complications to report to the physician, use of medical equipment, follow-up care, and referrals
▼ Documentation that the patient understands the teaching and that written instructions have been given to him or her
▼ Any exceptional details or unusual findings regarding the illness or present condition
▼ Condition of the patient at the time of discharge
▼ Description of status of wounds, dressings, drains, and tubes still in place
▼ Where to call and the phone numbers should further help be needed

EMERGENCIES
Nursing Actions in Case of Fire

Rescue any patients in immediate danger by removing them from the area.
Activate the fire alarm system and notify the telephone operator.
Contain the fire by closing doors and any open windows.
Extinguish the flames with an appropriate fire extinguisher.

Calling a "Code"

If the patient does not respond to your verbal call, follow basic cardiopulmonary resuscitation (CPR) guidelines:

▼ Turn on the call light, shout, or activate the bathroom call bell, which does not turn off until someone turns it off, as you begin to do the following:
- Shake the patient, shouting, "Are you all right?"
- Reposition to open airway.
- Look, listen, and feel for breath.
- Give two breaths if respiration is absent.
- Feel for a carotid pulse, or brachial pulse in an infant.
- Begin CPR (if pulseless), and continue until relieved.

Evaluating an ECG Rhythm Strip

When working with patients on telemetry or in the emergency department, you need to be able to do a basic evaluation of an electrocardiograph tracing (Figure 5-2). The following steps provide the needed data regarding the rate, rhythm, P-R interval duration of the QRS complex, and whether there are irregular beats.

▼ Obtain a 6-second strip (one with at least 10 large graph squares).
▼ Calculate the rate: Count the number of 0.2-second divisions between two consecutive QRS complexes and divide this into 300. This number is the heart rate.
▼ Measure the distance between the P waves. If the distance is the same, the rate is regular. Calculate the atrial rate by counting the

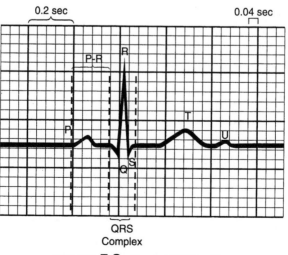

FIGURE 5-2 Normal ECG tracing.

number of small boxes between the P waves and dividing that number into 1500. This provides the atrial rate.

▼ Measure the P-R interval. Is it normal (0.12-0.20 s)? Does it vary?

▼ Measure the QRS duration. Is it normal (0.04-0.12 s)? Measure with calipers from R wave to R wave throughout the tracing to determine whether the rate is regular. Are there premature QRS complexes? Do all the QRS complexes look the same? Calculate the ventricular rate by counting the number of small squares between R waves and dividing that number into 1500. Are the atrial and ventricular rates the same? A rough calculation can be made by counting the number of complexes in a 6-second tracing and multiplying by 10. This gives the ventricular rate.

▼ Figure 5-3 shows the results of an analysis of a normal sinus rhythm.

Telemetry Monitoring

When placing the patient on cardiac telemetry monitoring, one of two leads is most commonly used with either two electrodes or three electrodes and a ground being attached to the patient (Figure 5-4).

Care and Observation during a Seizure

▼ Assist the patient to a lying position, move objects out of the way, and loosen any tight clothing.

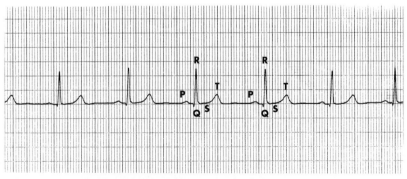

1. Rate between 50-100 bpm and regular.
2. P wave precedes each QRS complex; PR interval between 0.12-0.20 sec (3-5 small squares).
3. QRS duration between 0.04-0.12 sec (1-3 small squares).
4. QRS complexes have essentially the same shape.

FIGURE 5-3 Interpreting an electrocardiogram. (From Lewis SM, Heitkemper MM, Dirksen SR, O'Brien PG, Bucher L: *Medical-surgical nursing: assessment and management of clinical problems,* ed 7, St Louis, 2007, Mosby, p 856.)

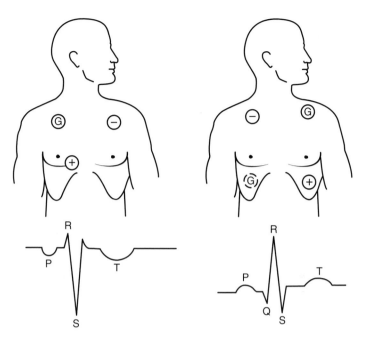

Placement of MCL₁ electrodes.　　Placement of lead II electrodes.

FIGURE 5-4 Placement of most commonly used telemetry leads. (Adapted from Hatchett R, Thompson D: *Cardiac nursing*, Philadelphia, 2002, Churchill Livingstone.)

▼ Do not restrain the patient.
▼ Place something soft under the head, if possible, such as a pillow, folded towel, or piece of clothing.
▼ Gently turn the head to the side to prevent aspiration of saliva.
▼ Do not force anything into the mouth; if the teeth are not clenched, place a soft object such as a washcloth between the teeth to protect the tongue.
▼ Note the time the seizure begins and ends.
▼ Note the progression of movements because this is important information for the physician.
▼ Call for assistance, but stay with the patient.
▼ Remember that respirations sometimes are irregular or cease during a seizure for a short period.
▼ Note if the patient becomes incontinent.
▼ Provide privacy if possible.
▼ Reassure the patient that you are there.
▼ After the seizure is over, reorient the patient, and tell him or her that a seizure has occurred.
▼ Record in detail all observations during the seizure.

MEASUREMENTS AND CONVERSIONS
Temperature Conversion

Celsius (Centigrade): 0	Fahrenheit: 32
36.0	96.8
36.5	97.7
37.0	98.6 (normal)
37.5	99.5
38.0	100.4
38.5	101.3
39.0	102.2
39.5	103.1
40.0	104.0
40.5	104.9
41.0	105.8
41.5	106.7
42.0	107.6

Convert Celsius readings to Fahrenheit by multiplying by 1.8 and adding 32. Convert Fahrenheit readings to Celsius by subtracting 32 and dividing by 1.8.

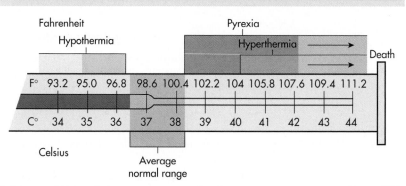

Celsius and Fahrenheit temperatures related to temperature ranges. (From Elkin et al: *Nursing interventions and clinical skills*, ed 3, St Louis, 2004, Mosby, p 268.)

Regular Clock Versus the 24-Hour Clock (Military Time)

Common Time	24-Hour Time	Common Time	24-Hour Time	Common Time	24-Hour Time
1:00 AM	0100	9:00 AM	0900	5:00 PM	1700
2:00 AM	0200	10:00 AM	1000	6:00 PM	1800
3:00 AM	0300	11:00 AM	1100	7:00 PM	1900
4:00 AM	0400	12:00 Noon	1200	8:00 PM	2000
5:00 AM	0500	1:00 PM	1300	9:00 PM	2100
6:00 AM	0600	2:00 PM	1400	10:00 PM	2200
7:00 AM	0700	3:00 PM	1500	11:00 PM	2300
8:00 AM	0800	4:00 PM	1600	12:00 (midnight)	2400

Apothecary and Metric Volume and Weight Equivalents

Weight Equivalents: Conversion

	Metric	Apothecary*
Gram (g)	Milligram (mg)	Grain (gr)
1	1000	15
0.5	500	7½
0.3	300 (325)	5
0.1	100	1½
0.06	60 (64)	1
0.03	30 (32)	½
0.015	15 (16)	¼
0.010	10	⅙
0.0006	0.6	⅟₁₀₀
0.0004	0.4	⅟₁₅₀
0.0003	0.3	⅟₂₀₀

*Apothecary measurements are not within recommended use but may occasionally be encountered.

Volume Equivalents: Liquid Conversion

30 mL	=	1 oz (fl ℥) = 2 tbsp (T) = 6 tsp = (t)
15 mL	=	½ oz = 1 T = 3t
1000 mL	=	1 quart (qt) = 1 liter (L)
500 mL	=	1 pint (pt)
5 mL	=	1 tsp (t)
4 mL	=	1 fl dr (fl D)
1 mL	=	15 (16) minims = 15 (16) drops (gtts)

From Kee J, Hayes E, McCuistion L: *Pharmacology: a nursing process approach*, ed 5, Philadelphia, 2006, Saunders. Reprinted with permission.

MOST COMMON LABORATORY TEST VALUES

All abnormal test values must be reported to the physician as soon as they are received.

Complete Blood Count (CBC)

	Conventional Units	S.I. Units
Cell counts		
Erythrocytes (RBCs)		
Male adults	4.6-6.2 million/mm^3	4.6-6.2 × 10^{12}/L
Female adults	4.2-5.4 million/mm^3	4.2-5.4 × 10^{12}/L
Children	4.5-5.1 million/mm^3	4.5-5.1 × 10^{12}/L
(varies with age)		

Complete Blood Count (CBC)—cont'd

	Conventional Units		S.I. Units
Leukocytes (WBCs)			
Total	4500-11,000/mm^3		4.5-11.0 × 10^9/L
Differential	*Percentage*	*Absolute*	
Myelocytes	0	0/mm^3	0/L
Band neutrophils	3-5	150-400/mm^3	150-400 × 10^6/L
Segmented	54-62	3,000-	3000-5800 × 10^6/L
neutrophils		5,800/mm^3	
Lymphocytes	25-33	1,500-3,000/mm^3	1500-3000 × 10^6/L
Monocytes	3-7	300-500/mm^3	300-500 × 10^6/L
Eosinophils	1-3	50-250/mm^3	50-250 × 10^6/L
Basophils	0-1	15-50/mm^3	15-50 × 10^6/L
Platelets	150,000-400,000/mm^3		150-350 × 10^9/L
Reticulocytes	25,000-75,000/mm^3		25-75 × 10^9/L
	(0.5-1.5% of erythrocytes)		
Hemoglobin			
Male adults	13.0-18.0 g/dL		8.1-11.2 mmol/L
Female adults	12.0-16.0 g/dL		7.4-9.9 mmol/L
Newborn	16.5-19.5 g/dL		10.2-12.1 mmol/L
Children (varies with age)	11.2-16.5 g/dL		7.0-10.2 mmol/L
Hemoglobin, fetal total	Less than 1%.0% of total		Less than 0.01
Hematocrit			of total
Male adults	40-54 mL/dL		0.40-0.54
Female adults	37-47 mL/dL		0.37-0.47
Newborn	49-54 mL/dL		0.49-0.54
Children (varies with age)	35-49 mL/dL		0.35-0.49
Corpuscular values of erythrocytes (values are for adults; in children, values vary with age)			
MCH (mean corpuscular hemoglobin)	26-34 pg/cell		26-34 pg/cell
MCV (mean corpuscular volume)	80-96 μm^3		80-96 fL
MCHC (mean corpuscular hemoglobin concentration)	32-36 g/dL		320-360 g/L

Adapted from Rakel RE, Bope ET, editors: *Conn's current therapy*, Philadelphia, 2006, Saunders. Reprinted with permission.

Routine Urinalysis

Component	Normal Values
Color	Pale yellow to deep amber
Opacity	Clear
Specific gravity	1.002-1.035
Osmolality	275-295 mOsm/L
pH	4.5-8

Routine Urinalysis—cont'd

Component	Normal Values
Glucose	Negative
Ketones	Negative
Protein	Negative
Bilirubin	Negative
Red blood cells	None to 3
White blood cells	None to 4
Bacteria	None
Casts	None
Crystals	None

From Black J, Hawks JH: *Medical-surgical nursing: clinical management for positive outcomes*, ed 7, Philadelphia, 2005, Saunders, p 97. Reprinted with permission.

Laboratory Values for an SMAC Test

	Conventional Units	S.I. Units
Electrolytes		
Sodium, serum	135-145 mEq/L	135-145 mmol/L
Potassium, serum	3.5-5.0 mEq/L	3.5-5.0 mmol/L
Chloride, serum	96-106 mEq/L	90-106 mmol/L
Calcium, serum	8.4-10.6 mg/dL	2.10-2.65 mmol/L
Chemical Values		
Glucose, serum (fasting)	70-115 mg/dL	3.9-6.4 mmol/L
Creatinine, serum	0.6-1.2 mg/dL	50-110 µmol/L
Uric acid, serum	2.4-7.0 mg/dL	143-416 µmol/L
Blood urea nitrogen (BUN), serum	11-23 mg/dL	8.0-16.4 µmol/L
Bilirubin, total serum	0.3-1.1 mg/dL	5.1-19 mmol/L
Carbon dioxide, serum	24-31 mEq/L	24-31 mmol/L
Total protein, serum	6.0-8.0 g/dL	60-80 g/L
Albumin, serum	3.5-5.2 g/dL	35-52 g/L
Globulin, serum	2.5 g % of protein	
A/G ratio	1.5:1 to 2.5:1	
Alanine aminotransferase (ALT), serum (SGPT)	1-45 U/L	1-45 U/L
Aspartate aminotransferase (AST), serum (SGOT)	1-36 U/L	1-36 U/L
Cholesterol		
Total cholesterol, serum	<200 mg/dL	<5.20 mmol/L
LDL, serum	60-180 mg/dL	600-1800 mg/L
HDL, serum	30-80 mg/dL	300-800 mg/L
Triglycerides, serum	40-150 mg/dL	0.4-1.5 g/L

Normal Range Values for Arterial Blood Gases*

pH	7.35-7.45
$Paco_2$	35-45 mm Hg
Hco_3	22-26 mEq/L
Pao_2	80%-100%

*Values may vary slightly among laboratories.

MEDICATION ADMINISTRATION
Abbreviations Related to Medication Administration

mL	=	milliliter
fl oz	=	fl ℥
g, Gm, G, GM	=	gram
gr	=	grain
gtt	=	drop
kg	=	kilogram
mcg	=	microgram
mEq	=	milliequivalent
mg	=	milligram
l, L	=	liter
s̄s̄	=	one-half
T, tbsp	=	tablespoon
t, tsp	=	teaspoon
<	=	less than
>	=	greater than
PO, po, os	=	by mouth
AC, ac	=	before meals
PC, pc	=	after meals
c̄	=	with
s̄	=	without
Bid, bid	=	twice a day
Tid, tid	=	three times a day
Qid, qid	=	four times a day
q4, 6, 8h	=	every 4, 6, 8 hours
PRN	=	whenever necessary
NPO	=	nothing by mouth
STAT	=	immediately
IM	=	intramuscularly
IV	=	intravenously
subcut.	=	subcutaneously
SL, subl	=	sublingual
IVPB	=	intravenous piggyback
KVO	=	keep vein open

From Kee J, Hayes E, McCuistion L: *Pharmacology: a nursing process approach*, ed 5, Philadelphia, 2006, Saunders. Reprinted with permission.

Five Rights of Medication Administration

▼ **Give the right medication:** Check the prescriber's order, and check the label with the medication administration record three times.

▼ **Give the right dose:** Check the prescriber's order, check the dosage on the medication label three times, and calculate the correct amount to give per the order.

▼ **Give the medication at the right time:** Check the prescriber's order, and check the date and time on the medication administration record order three times. Check the expiration date of the medication.

▼ **Give the medication by the right route:** Check the prescriber's order and verify the route of administration three times on the medication administration record.

▼ **Give the medication to the right patient:** Check the armband name and number with the medication administration record sheet just before administering the drug, and ask the patient to state his or her name. Each unit dose drug should be checked with the medication administration record, verifying each of the first four rights:
  - As the medication is taken from the patient's drawer.
  - As the medication is placed, still in its package, in a paper cup or on a small tray.
  - Just before opening the package to administer the dose to the patient.

Safety Guidelines to Prevent Medication Errors*

When preparing to administer medications:

▼ Ask yourself why this drug is prescribed for this patient. Know the drug, the patient, and all of the patient's medical conditions.

▼ Before preparing medications, verify which patients are NPO or off the unit.

▼ Verify that the medication orders on the MAR/Kardex have been checked against the prescriber's orders.

▼ If the patient is a child or an older adult, review the special precautions to be considered.

▼ Become familiar with the "high alert drug list" from your facility's pharmacy. Be extra careful when administering a drug that is on this list. Be aware of look-alike and sound-alike drugs.

▼ Become familiar with the list of abbreviations that are no longer to be used and ask for verification from the prescriber as to what is intended by the abbreviation if it appears in an order.

▼ Plan ahead and do not rush when preparing medications for administration.

▼ Prepare medications for administration in as distraction-free an environment as possible.

---

*Adapted from deWit S: *Fundamental concepts and skills for nursing,* ed 2, Philadelphia, 2005, Elsevier.

▼ Follow the five rights of medication administration every time you prepare and give medications.

▼ Check each medication with the order thoroughly three times before giving it to the patient.

▼ Ask before crushing a drug if you do not know whether it can be safely administered after crushing.

▼ Clarify with the prescriber any illegible writing in a drug order.

▼ Do not administer a drug if it is not clearly and correctly labeled with name and amount of the drug contained.

▼ Do not unwrap a unit dose drug before you are at the patient's bedside and ready to administer the medication.

▼ Check any questionable order or unfamiliar drug or dosage with the pharmacist.

▼ If an ordered drug dosage seems odd, question it and check the order with the pharmacist or physician.

▼ Check pertinent laboratory values and assess for side effects of the drug before giving the next dose.

▼ If a dosage calculation has to be made, have the calculation repeated by another nurse and compare the result.

▼ Review the patient's MAR for any possible drug interactions.

▼ Determine if the patient is receiving more than one drug with the same action. If so, question the order.

▼ Ask another nurse to double-check the order and dose you are going to give of any high-risk drug such as IV potassium, heparin, IV cardiac drugs, and insulins.

▼ Keep the drug in its original container. Discard leftover portions of unused medication from single-dose packages.

▼ Whenever multiple tablets or vials are needed to prepare a single dose of medication, check with the pharmacist to verify the amount is correct per the order.

▼ Become aware of drugs with similar names and carefully check the original order and why the patient is receiving the drug before administering it.

▼ Question an excessive dosage increase in a patient's medication.

▼ Be familiar with every drug you administer. Look it up if you can't remember the information you need to safely administer it.

▼ Date multiple-dose medication vials as you open them.

At the time of medication administration to the patient:

▼ Use two patient identifiers. Verify the name and number on the patient's armband with the information on the MAR each time you administer medications to the patient.

▼ Check the medication administration record and the chart for noted allergies and question the patient before administering medications.

▼ Check each drug at the bedside with the patient's MAR before administering the medication.

▼ If the patient questions the drug or dose you are about to give, stop and check the situation.

▼ Sign that a medication has been given only after the patient has received it.

▼ Do not leave a medication dose at the patient's bedside.

▼ Document only after the patient has actually taken the medication.

Working with the patient for error prevention:

▼ Teach the patient about the drugs he or she is taking and the importance of proper identification of the patient before a drug is taken.

▼ Familiarize the patient with the color and shape of each medication, but consider that generic forms of the drug may differ. Instruct the patient to ask the pharmacist if a refill looks different than the last one.

▼ Obtain a complete drug history from the patient, including herbals, over-the-counter medications, and supplements.

If a medication error does occur, always report it.

Check Those Lab Tests!

When preparing to administer medications, you should know the laboratory test values relative to the action or potential adverse effects of each drug. For some drugs you will be checking to see if the medication is effective; for others, checking indicates if the drug is at a therapeutic level in the patient's body. Many drugs can affect kidney function, liver function, or bone marrow/blood cell function, and laboratory tests are checked to verify whether adverse effects are occurring. Checking your patient's lab values first thing during the shift will save you time later. You will not always find the laboratory test data you are seeking, but it is your responsibility to check. Become familiar with the laboratory test values that should be checked when giving various medications. Here is a list of common medications, or types of medication, and the test values to be checked. This is not a complete list. Check your drug handbook for other specific test values that should be checked for a particular medication.

Medication	Laboratory Test Value to Check
Digoxin (Lanoxin)	Serum digoxin; K^+
Lasix	K^+
Procainamide	Serum level
Heparin	aPPT
Warfarin (Coumadin)	INR, PT
Antibiotics	CBC
Tobramycin	Serum peak and trough levels
Gentamicin	Liver functions—AST, ALT, bilirubin
Vancomycin	Kidney functions—BUN, creatinine
Chloramphenicol	LDH, alkaline phosphatase
Amikacin	Therapeutic level; BUN, creatinine

Continued

Medication	Laboratory Test Value to Check
Anticonvulsants	Specific drug serum level
	CBC, AST, ALT, bilirubin, BUN, creatinine
Theophylline, aminophylline (bronchodilators)	Serum theophylline level
Albuterol	ABGs
Antihypertensives	CBC, electrolytes
NSAIDs, acetaminophen, ibuprofen	CBC, liver functions—AST, ALT; kidney functions—BUN, creatinine
Hypoglycemics, insulins	Serum glucose, fingerstick glucose
Cortisone, corticosteroids	K+, CBC, serum glucose
Cholesterol-lowering statins	Cholesterol, HDL, LDL, triglycerides, AST, ALT, CPK
Iron preparations	CBC, HgB, Hct

Choosing the Correct Needle Size

The larger the number of the gauge, the smaller the needle is.

For	Use
Intradermal injection	
Intradermal skin test	27 gauge, ½ in
Subcutaneous injection	
Allergy injection	27 gauge, ½ in or ⅜ in
Immunization (some)	25 gauge, ⅝ in
Intramuscular injection	
Thin solutions	23-25 gauge, 1 to 1½ in*
Antibiotic	22 gauge, 1 to 1½ in*
Oil-based solution	21 gauge, 1 to 1½ in*

*Length depends on size of patient and the injection site chosen; larger patients need a longer needle to reach the proper depth.

Guidelines for Insulin Administration

▼ Check all insulin orders with the physician's order sheet.

▼ Verify the patient's current blood sugar level per glucometer reading or lab work. Assess the patient for signs of hyperglycemia or hypoglycemia. Symptoms of **hyperglycemia** include nausea; vomiting; abdominal cramps; fatigue; increased thirst; increased urination; increased hunger followed by anorexia; weakness; dry mouth; acetone breath; and rapid, deep respirations. Signs of **hypoglycemia** include sweating; cold; clammy skin; feelings of numbness in fingers, toes, around mouth; rapid heartbeat; headache; nervousness; shakiness; faintness; slurred speech; hunger; vision changes; unsteady gait; weakness. Obtain permission to recheck blood sugar by glucometer.

▼ Administer insulin as close to the time ordered as possible, but consider when a meal will be served.

▼ Shake or gently roll and invert the bottle to mix and ensure even drug particle distribution before withdrawing the solution from the vial.

▼ Check date on vial to be certain the insulin is in-date.

▼ When mixing regular and longer-acting insulin, put air into the longer-acting insulin vial, then put air into the regular insulin and draw up the correct amount of the regular insulin; draw up the exact amount of the longer-acting insulin last.

▼ Always have another nurse verify the type and dosage of each insulin ordered as you prepare the injection.

▼ Use only an insulin syringe (insulin syringes are measured in units of insulin).

▼ Inject at a 45- to 60-degree angle.

▼ Rotate injection sites to prevent lipodystrophy. Do not massage the site after injection. Use one site daily for 1 week, then rotate to a new site. Keep a record of injection sites. Sites within an area should be $1\frac{1}{2}$ inches apart. Abdominal sites are preferred for consistent absorption.

▼ If patient gives his or her own insulin at home and is able to administer it in the hospital, allow the opportunity to do so.

▼ Never give any type but regular insulin by IV infusion.

▼ Watch for signs of hypoglycemia around the time that the insulin given is expected to peak (see Insulins and Their Actions later in this chapter). Give oral carbohydrate snack if symptoms occur and blood sugar reading is low. Milk and crackers, or 4 ounces of orange juice, are commonly given.

▼ Report hypoglycemic reactions to the staff nurse and your instructor immediately.

▼ Remember that only regular insulin can be given IV.

▼ Continue to monitor the patient.

Hypoglycemia Versus Hyperglycemia

	Hypoglycemia (<60 mg/dL)	Hyperglycemia (>250 mg/dL)
Cause	▼ Too much insulin	▼ Too little insulin
	▼ Skipped or delayed meals	▼ Overeating
		▼ Emotional stress
	▼ Too much exercise	▼ Illness, infection, stroke, heart attack, pregnancy
		▼ Ketoacidosis
Early symptoms	▼ Sweating, shaking, weakness	▼ Excessive thirst
	▼ Headache, dizziness	▼ Frequent urination
	▼ Hunger	▼ Fatigue, weakness
Late symptoms	▼ Numbness of lips/tongue	▼ Nausea, vomiting, abdominal pain
	▼ Difficulty concentrating	▼ Flushed, dry skin
	▼ Irritability, mood change	▼ Fruity breath, drowsiness, lethargy
	▼ Blurred vision, pallor	▼ Loss of appetite, general aching

Continued

Hypoglycemia Versus Hyperglycemia—cont'd

Hypoglycemia (<60 mg/dL)	Hyperglycemia (>250 mg/dL)
▼ If untreated: seizures, coma	▼ If untreated: labored breathing, coma

Adapted from *Mosby's nursing PDQ for LPN,* St Louis, 2005, Mosby, p 57.

Sites for Intramuscular (IM) and Subcutaneous (subcut) Injections

See Figure 5-5 for intramuscular and subcutaneous injection sites.

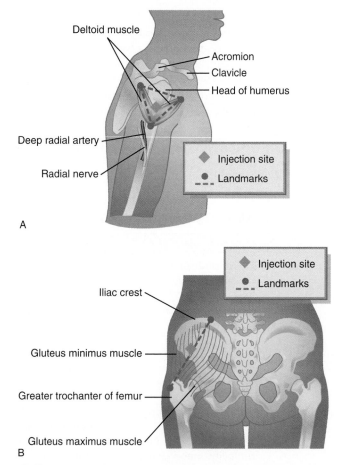

FIGURE 5-5   Intramuscular and subcutaneous injection sites: **(A)** deltoid, **(B)** dorso-gluteal, **(C)** ventrogluteal, **(D)** vastus lateralis, and **(E)** rectus femoris. (From Kee J, Hayes E, McCuistion L: *Pharmacology: a nursing process approach*, ed 5, Philadelphia, 2006, Saunders, p 38.)

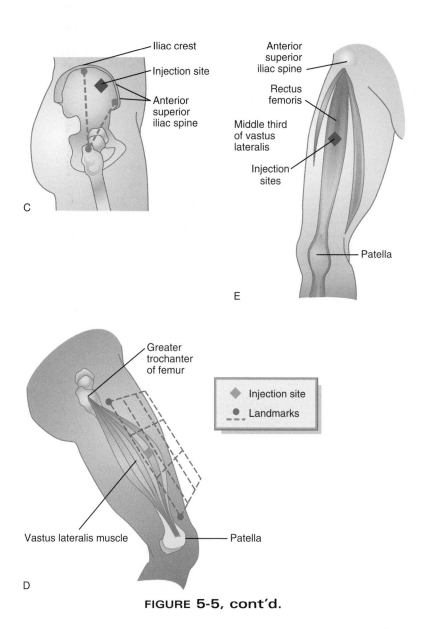

FIGURE 5-5, cont'd.

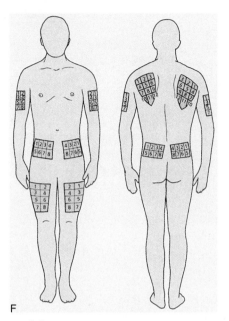

F

FIGURE 5-5, cont'd   Intramuscular and subcutaneous injection sites: **(F)** rotation of sites for subcutaneous injections.

Dosage and Solution Calculation Formulas

Drug Calculations: Basic Formula

$$\frac{D \text{ (desire)}}{H \text{ (on hand)}} \times V \text{ (vehicle, drug form)}$$

Example:

Order: amoxicillin 100 mg, po, q6h
Available: amoxicillin 250 mg/5 mL

$$\frac{D}{H} \times V = \frac{100 \text{ mg}}{250 \text{ mg}} \times 5 \text{ mL}$$

$$= \frac{500}{250} = 2 \text{ mL amoxicillin}$$

Dosage and Solution Calculation Formulas—cont'd

Drug Calculations: Ratio and Proportion

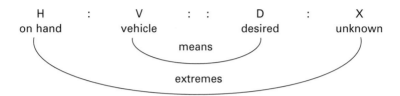

Example:

Order: amoxicillin 100 mg, po, q6h
Available: amoxicillin 250 mg/5 mL

H	:	V	: :	D	:	X
250 mg	:	5 mL	: :	100 mg	:	X mL

$$250 \text{ X} = 500$$
$$\text{X} = 2 \text{ mL amoxicillin}$$

Body Weight (Kilograms)

To change pounds to kilograms, divide by 2.2.

Example:

Change 44 pounds to kg

$$44 \div 2.2 = 20 \text{ kg}$$
Dosage/kg/day = dosage/day
(dosage × kg = dose/day)

Example:

Order: drug 6 mg/kg/day in four divided doses

6 mg × 20 kg × 1 day = 120 mg/day
120 ÷ 4 = 30 mg per dose

From Kee J, Hayes E, McCuistion L: *Pharmacology: a nursing process approach,* ed 5, Philadelphia, 2006, Saunders, p 72. Reprinted with permission.

Insulins and Their Actions

Insulin	Description and Route	Onset of Action	Peak Action	Duration of Action
Rapid-Acting				
Lispro (Humalog)	Clear, subcut	5 min	0.5-1 h	2-4 h
Apidra (insulin-glulisine)	Clear, subcut	5 min	55 min	6-8 h
Aspart (NovoLog)	Clear, subcut	10-15 min	1-3 h	3-5 h
Regular	Clear, subcut or IV	10 min-1 h	2-4 h	8-10 h
Humulin R	Clear, subcut or IV	10 min-1 h	2-4 h	6-8 h
Intermediate-Acting				
NPH protamine	Cloudy, subcut	1-2 h	6-12 h	18-24 h
Humulin N	Cloudy, subcut	1-2 h	8-12 h	18-24 h
Humulin L	Cloudy, subcut	1-2 h	8-12 h	18-28 h
Long-Acting				
Glargine (Lantus)	Cloudy, subcut	1.1 h	5 h	24 h
Levemir	Cloudy, subcut	2-4 h	None	20-24 h
Combinations				
Humulin 70/30 (NPH 70%, regular 30%)	Cloudy, subcut	0.5 h	4-8 h	22-24 h
Humulin 50/50 (NPH 50%, regular 50%)	Cloudy, subcut	0.5 h	4-8 h	24 h
Humalog 75/25 (Lispro protamine 75%, Lispro 25%)	Cloudy, subcut	15 min	0.5-6 h	20-24 h

IV, intravenous; *subcut*, subcutaneous.
Adapted from Kee JL, Hayes ER, McCuistion L: *Pharmacology: a nursing process approach*, ed 5, Philadelphia, 2006, Saunders, p 848. Reprinted with permission.

Guidelines for Digitalis Therapy

Digitalis is given to strengthen myocardial muscle action and slow the heart rate. Drug toxicity occurs frequently with this drug. **Early signs of toxicity** include anorexia, diarrhea, headache, confusion, fatigue, irritability, drowsiness, and halos around lights or green or yellow vision. **Further signs of toxicity** include cardiac arrythmia, particularly bradycardia, depression, and convulsion. **A below-normal serum potassium level predisposes to digitalis toxicity.**

Nursing Considerations

▼ Auscultate the apical pulse for 60 seconds to detect changes in rate or rhythm.

▼ If the heart rate is less than 60 or more than 100, check the physician's orders for a notation as to whether the dose should be given or if it should be withheld until the physician has been notified. Assess for other signs of toxicity before calling the physician (dose is held if toxicity is present).

▼ Check the last laboratory test level of digitalis and the last serum potassium before administering the dose. Assess for signs of hypokalemia: muscle weakness, fatigue, anorexia, confusion, weak pulse, nausea.

▼ Assess total medication regimen to determine possible interactions of digitalis with other drugs.

▼ If the patient is taking both digitalis and a diuretic that is not potassium sparing, potassium supplementation should be administered.

Patient Teaching for Digitalis Therapy

▼ Digitalis preparations should be taken at the same time each day.

▼ Check the pulse for a full minute before taking each dose.

▼ Report signs of digitalis toxicity; pay attention to early signs.

▼ Report any new irregular rhythm or abnormal pulse rate to the physician.

▼ Watch for signs of potassium depletion (hypokalemia). Teach the signs.

▼ Do not skip doses of prescribed potassium supplement.

▼ If a digitalis dose is missed, do not take an extra dose without consulting the physician.

▼ Keep follow-up appointments with the physician.

Guidelines for Steroid (Cortisone) Therapy

▼ Once-a-day steroid doses are given between 7:00 AM and 8:00 AM for best results because this is when the body normally releases these hormones.

▼ Check for possible interactions with other drugs the patient is receiving.

▼ Insulin dosages may need to be adjusted when the patient is receiving steroids.

▼ Administer oral steroids with food or milk to minimize gastric irritation.

▼ Patients who are NPO and are receiving parenteral steroids should be monitored for gastric bleeding. Medications to protect the gastric mucosa are usually given concurrently.

▼ Do not omit steroid dosages. If a dose has been inadvertently skipped, consult the physician.

▼ If the patient has been receiving steroids for 1 week or longer, the dosage must be tapered slowly rather than discontinuing the drug abruptly.

▼ Observe for infection and protect the patient from exposure to infection while receiving steroids. Steroids can mask infection and sometimes suppress the immune system.

▼ Assess for potassium imbalances and glucose imbalances.

▼ Increase calcium intake. Teach patient on long-term steroid therapy measures to help prevent osteoporosis.

▼ Encourage regular eye examination when the patient is on long-term therapy; steroids can cause cataracts and glaucoma.

▼ Assess for Cushing syndrome symptoms: moon face, buffalo hump, hirsutism, edema.

▼ Observe for side effects of steroid therapy: nausea, abdominal pain, hypertension, pathologic fractures, osteoporosis, delayed wound healing, headache, mood changes, insomnia, dizziness on standing.

Guidelines for Anticoagulant Therapy

Your patient may receive heparin by continuous intravenous infusion, intermittent intravenous injection, or subcutaneous injection. Consider the following points:

▼ Protamine sulfate is the antidote for heparin overdose and should be kept on hand on the unit.

▼ The effectiveness of heparin therapy is judged by the extension of usual clotting time to 2 to 2.5 times normal (approximately 60 to 70 seconds). The activated partial thromboplastin time (APTT) or partial thromboplastin time (PTT) is used to determine the clotting time. The result should be no more than 2 to 2.5 times the control time. The test should be done before therapy is begun and then monitored periodically depending on how much heparin the patient is receiving and whether it is being given intravenously or by injection.

▼ **All heparin dosages should be checked with another nurse as they are prepared.**

▼ Heparin subcutaneous injections are given in the abdominal fat at least 2 inches from the umbilicus in the area between the iliac crests.

▼ Do not aspirate before injecting the heparin because this causes tissue trauma and bruising.

▼ Wait 10 to 15 seconds after injecting before removing the needle.

▼ Do not massage the area because this causes increased bruising.

▼ Ice may be applied for 5 minutes to prevent bruising if this is a problem for the patient.

▼ Rotate the injection site from side to side.

▼ The patient receiving heparin by continuous intravenous infusion should be placed on a special mattress to decrease bruising.

▼ Monitor the patient closely for signs of increased bleeding or hemorrhage such as bloody urine (hematuria); dark, tarry stools (melana); bleeding of surgical wounds; bleeding gums; nosebleeds (epistaxis); hematomas; bloody sputum; bruising (ecchymosis); increased vaginal bleeding; neurologic changes; and signs and symptoms of hypovolemic shock.

Patients who have been treated with heparin are often started on warfarin sodium (Coumadin) orally before the heparin is discontinued. This is done because it takes 3 days for the warfarin levels in the blood to build up to an effective anticoagulant level.

▼ Warfarin therapy's effectiveness is judged by the prothrombin time (PT) test. The result should be no more than 2 to 2.5 times the control value (usually 12 to 14 seconds). Prothrombin time international normalized ratio (INR) is therapeutic from 2.0 to 3.0. When intracoronary stents or recurrent systemic emboli are treated with warfarin, the INR is kept between 3.0 and 4.5.

▼ The antidote for warfarin overdosage is vitamin K by injection.

Patient Teaching for Anticoagulant Therapy

▼ Caution the patient not to take aspirin, NSAIDs, or other salicylates while receiving anticoagulants.

▼ Avoid situations that could cause injury and bleeding, including contact sports. An electric razor may be used rather than a safety razor. Use a soft toothbrush, and avoid vigorous nose blowing.

▼ Many medications interact with warfarin; consult the physician regarding the possible interaction with other medications and supplements.

▼ Keep the amount of green vegetables containing vitamin K consistent in the diet.

▼ Limit alcohol intake.

▼ Take the medication at the same time each day.

▼ Inform all physicians and dentists that the patient is on an anticoagulant.

▼ Wear an ID band stating that an anticoagulant is being taken.

▼ If bleeding occurs, apply pressure for 5 to 10 minutes and call the physician.

▼ Schedule follow-up tests to determine effect of anticoagulant.

Reference Values for Therapeutic Drug Monitoring

Therapeutic Test	Range	Proprietary Test Toxic Levels	Names
Antibiotics			
Amikacin, serum	25-30 mcg/mL	Peak >35 mcg/mL Trough >10 mcg/mL	Amikin
Chloramphenicol, serum	10-20 mcg/mL	>25 mcg/mL	Chloromycetin
Gentamicin, serum	5-10 mcg/mL	Peak >10 mcg/mL Trough >2 mcg/mL	Garamycin
Tobramycin, serum	5-10 mcg/mL	Peak >10 mcg/mL Trough >2 mcg/mL	Nebcin
Vancomycin, serum	5-35 mcg/mL	Peak >40 mcg/mL Trough >10 mcg/mL	

Continued

Reference Values for Therapeutic Drug Monitoring—cont'd

Therapeutic Test	Range	Proprietary Test Toxic Levels	Names
Anticonvulsants			
Carbamazepine, serum	5-12 mcg/mL	>15 mcg/mL	Tegretol
Ethosuximide, serum	40-100 mcg/mL	>150 mcg/mL	Zarontin
Phenobarbital, serum	15-40 mcg/mL	40-100 mcg/mL (vary widely)	Luminal
Phenytoin, serum	10-20 mcg/mL	>20 mcg/mL	Dilantin
Primidone, serum	5-12 mcg/mL	>15 mcg/mL	Mysoline
Valproic acid, serum	50-100 mcg/mL	>100 mcg/mL	Depakene
Analgesics			
Acetaminophen, serum	10-20 mcg/mL	>250 mcg/mL	Tylenol Datril
Salicylate, serum	100-250 mcg/mL	>300 mcg/mL	
Bronchodilators			
Theophylline, serum (aminophylline)	10-20 mcg/mL	>20 mcg/mL	Theo-Dur
Cardiovascular Drugs			
Amiodarone, serum (obtain specimen more than 8 h after last dose)	1-2 mcg/mL	>2 mcg/mL	Cordarone
Digitoxin, serum (specimen must be obtained 12 to 24 h after last dose)	15-25 ng/mL	>35 ng/mL	Crystodigin
Digoxin, serum (specimen must be obtained 12 to 24 h after last dose)	0.8-2.0 ng/mL	>2.4 ng/mL	Lanoxin
Disopyramide, serum	2-5 mcg/mL	>7 mcg/mL	Norpace
Flecainide	0.2-1.0 ng/mL	>1 ng/mL	Tambocor
Lidocaine, serum	1.5-5.0 mcg/mL	>6 mcg/mL	Xylocaine
Mexilitine	0.7-2.0 ng/mL	>2 ng/mL	Mexitil
Procainamide, serum (measured as procainamide ++ N-acetyl-procainamide)	4-10 mcg/mL 8-30 mcg/mL	>12 mcg/mL >30 mcg/mL	Pronestyl
Propranolol, serum	50-100 ng/mL	Variable	Inderal

Reference Values for Therapeutic Drug Monitoring—cont'd

Therapeutic Test	Range	Proprietary Test Toxic Levels	Names
Quinidine, serum	2-5 mcg/mL	>6 mcg/mL	Cardioquin Quinaglute
Tocainide	4-10 ng/mL	>10 ng/mL	Tonogard
Psychopharmacologic Drugs			
Amitriptyline, serum (measured as amitriptyline + nortriptyline)	120-150 ng/mL	>500 ng mL	Elavil Endep Entrafon Limbitrol Triavil
Bupropion	25-100 ng/mL	Not applicable	Wellbutrin
Desipramine, serum (measured as desipramine ++ imipramine)	150-300 ng/mL	>500 ng/mL	Norpramin Petrofrane
Imipramine, serum (measured as imipramine ++ desipramine)	125-250 ng/mL	>400 ng/mL	Janimine Presamin Tofranil
Lithium, serum (obtain specimen 12 h after last dose)	0.6-1.5 mEq/L	>2.0 mEq/L	Lithobid
Nortriptyline, serum	50-150 ng/mL	>500 ng/mL	Aventyl Pamelor

Adapted from Rakel RE, Bope ET, editors: *Conn's current therapy*, Philadelphia, 2006, Elsevier, pp 1496-1497. Reprinted with permission.

Calculating Intravenous Flow Rates

IV Flow Rate: Continuous—Method I

Amount of fluid ÷ hours to administer = mL/h

$$\frac{mL/h \times gtts/mL \text{ (IV set)}}{60 \text{ min/h}} = gtts/min$$

Example:
Order: 1000 mL, D_5 ½ NS in 8 h
IV set: Macrodrip: 10 gtts/mL

1000 mL ÷ 8 h = 125 mL/h

$$\frac{125 \text{ mL/h} \times \overset{1}{10} \text{ gtts/mL}}{\underset{6}{60} \text{ min/h}} = 21 \text{ gtts/min}$$

IV Flow Rate: Intermittent—Volumetric Pump

$$\text{Amount of solution} \div \frac{\text{min to administer}}{60 \text{ min/h}} = \text{mL/h}$$

Order: Administer 5 mL of drug solution in 100 mL of D_5W in 45 min

$$105 \text{ mL} \div \frac{45 \text{ min}}{60 \text{ min/h}} \text{ (invert divisor and multiply)}$$

$$= 105 \times \frac{\overset{4}{\cancel{60}}}{\underset{3}{\cancel{45}}} = 140 \text{ mL/h}$$

Set volumetric pump at 140 mL/h to deliver 105 mL in 45 min

IV Flow Rate: Intermittent—Secondary Sets: Buretrol and Add-a-Line

$$\frac{\text{Amount of solution} \times \text{gtts/mL (set)}}{\text{Min to administer}} = \text{gtts/min}$$

Order: Administer 5 mL of drug solution in 50 mL of D_5W in 30 min
IV set: Buretrol (60 gtts/mL)

$$\frac{55 \text{ mL} \times \overset{2}{\cancel{60}} \text{ gtts}}{\underset{1}{\cancel{30}} \text{ min}} = 110 \text{ gtts/min}$$

IV Flow Rate: Continuous—Method II

$$\frac{\text{Amount of fluid} \times \text{gtts/mL (IV set)}}{\text{H to administer} \times \text{min/h (60)}} = \text{gtts/min}$$

Example:

Order: 1000 mL of D_5W in 10 h
IV set: Microdrip: 60 gtts/mL

$$\frac{\overset{100}{\cancel{1000}} \text{ mL} \times \overset{1}{\cancel{60}} \text{ gtts/mL}}{\underset{1}{\cancel{10}} \text{ h} \times \underset{1}{\cancel{60}} \text{ min/h}} = 100 \text{ gtts/min}$$

From Kee J, Hayes E, McCuistion L: *Pharmacology: a nursing process approach*, ed 5, Philadelphia, 2006, Saunders. Reprinted with permission.

Intravenous Flow Rate Chart

Administration Sets Delivering 10 drops (gtts)/mL

Amount to be infused	1000 mL	1000 mL	1000 mL	1000 mL
Time of infusion	12 h	10 h	8 h	6 h
Drops/minute of flow	14 gtts	17 gtts	21 gtts	28 gtts

Administration Sets Delivering 15 drops (gtts)/mL

Amount to be infused	1000 mL	1000 mL	1000 mL	1000 mL
Time of infusion	12 h	10 h	8 h	6 h
Drops/minute of flow	21 gtts	25 gtts	31 gtts	42 gtts

Administration Sets Delivering 20 drops (gtts)/mL

Amount to be infused	1000 mL	1000 mL	1000 mL	1000 mL
Time of infusion	12 h	10 h	8 h	6 h
Drops/minute of flow	28 gtts	33 gtts	42 gtts	56 gtts

Microdrip Administration Sets Delivering 60 drops (gtts)/mL

Amount to be infused	250 mL	250 mL	500 mL	1000 mL
Time of infusion	24 h	12 h	12 h	24 h
Drops/minute of flow	10 gtts	21 gtts	42 gtts	42 gtts

Administration Sets Delivering 10 drops (gtts)/mL

Amount to be infused	50 mL	50 mL	50 mL
Time of infusion	20 min	30 min	60 min
Rate of flow (drops/min)	25 gtts	17 gtts	8 gtts

Administration Sets Delivering 15 drops (gtts)/mL

Amount to be infused	50 mL	50 mL	50 mL
Time of infusion	20 min	30 min	60 min
Rate of flow (drops/min)	38 gtts	25 gtts	12 gtts

Administration Sets Delivering 20 drops (gtts)/mL

Amount to be infused	50 mL	50 mL	50 mL
Time of infusion	20 min	30 min	60 min
Rate of flow (drops/min)	50 gtts	33 gtts	17 gtts

Administration Sets Delivering 60 drops (gtts)/mL (Microdrip)

Amount to be infused	50 mL	100 mL	250 mL
Time of infusion	2 h	8 h	6 h
Rate of flow (drops/min)	25 gtts	12 gtts	42 gtts

Calculation of Intravenous Intake

Start with the amount that was in the intravenous container at the beginning of the shift. If that entire amount infuses and a new container is
hung, note the amount that infused from the old container on the shift
I&O sheet under "IV intake."

Next, at the end of the shift, note how much of the solution in the new
container hung during the shift has infused. Draw a line and initial it
with the time at that point on the container. Write the amount infused on
the shift I&O sheet under "IV intake." Add the two amounts together to
obtain the total IV intake for the shift.

To calculate the amount left to count in the IV container (for the next
shift), subtract the amount infused from the new container from the total
volume hung.

Example:

	Count	Infused
Count at beginning of shift	450 mL	
New solution added at 11:30 AM	1000 mL	450 mL
Amount infused at 2:00 PM		325 mL
Amount left to count at end of shift	675 mL	
Total amount of IV intake		775 mL

IV Site Placement

▼ Identify suitable vein for placement of IV catheter or needle. The cephalic,
basilic, and median cubital veins are preferred in adults (Figure 5-6).

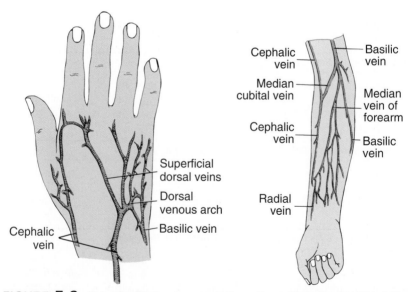

FIGURE 5-6 Veins for IV site placement. (From Perry AG, Potter PA, Elkin MK:
Nursing interventions and clinical skills, ed 3, St Louis, 2004, Mosby, p 679.)

▼ Use the most distal site in the nondominant arm, if possible. Choose a site that will least interfere with activities of daily living (ADLs).

▼ Clip arm hair with scissors if site has considerable hair.

▼ Place extremity in dependent position if possible.

▼ Place the tourniquet 4 to 6 inches above the chosen site. Do not apply tourniquet too tightly; check for radial pulse, indicating good blood flow distal to tourniquet.

▼ Release tourniquet temporarily and prepare all equipment. Replace tourniquet when ready to perform the puncture.

▼ Measures to increase venous distention include lightly tapping over the vein, stroking the extremity from distal to proximal below the proposed venipuncture site, having patient open and close the fist and then leaving it closed, applying moistened warm washcloth to site for several minutes, and dangling the extremity for several minutes.

▼ Follow correct procedure for cleansing the site and insertion of the catheter or needle. Always wear latex gloves when inserting an IV catheter or needle.

Characteristics of Commonly Used Intravenous Fluids

Solution	Tonicity	Calories	Use
0.9% saline (0.9% NS)	Isotonic	0	Fluid replacement, treatment of metabolic acidosis in presence of fluid loss, correction of sodium depletion; used before and after blood transfusion
0.45% saline (0.45% NS)	Hypotonic	0	Electrolyte replacement of sodium and chloride
5% dextrose in water (D_5W)	Isotonic	170	Treatment of hypovolemia
10% dextrose in water ($D_{10}W$)	Hypertonic	340	Nutrient and electrolyte replacement
5% dextrose in 0.9% saline (D_5NS 0.9%)	Hypertonic	170	Treatment of circulatory insufficiency; fluid re-replacement
5% dextrose in 0.45% water ($D_5\frac{1}{2}NS$)	Hypertonic	170	Maintenance of body fluids with nutrients and for treatment of fluid volume deficit
10% dextrose in 0.9% saline ($D_{10}NS$ 0.9%)	Hypertonic	340	Nutrient and electrolyte replacement (sodium and chloride)
Ringer's lactate Hartmann's solution (RL)	Isotonic	0	Extracellular fluid replacement for loss due to vomiting, diarrhea, or severe diuresis

Continued

Characteristics of Commonly Used Intravenous Fluids—cont'd

Solution	Tonicity	Calories	Use
5% dextrose in lactated Ringer's (D₅RL)	Hypertonic	170	Electrolyte replacement plus nutrient
Ringer's solution	Isotonic	0	Replaces sodium without increasing chloride levels

Setting up a "Piggyback" Minibag Medication

1. Check the medication with the order.
2. Verify that the medication is compatible with the main IV solution and its additives.
3. Remove the secondary (piggyback) tubing from its package and close the roller clamp.
4. Spike the piggyback medication container.
5. Squeeze the drip chamber and open the roller clamp to prime the tubing, keeping the connector sterile.
6. Recheck the medication with the order or MAR.
7. Take the medication to the patient and perform the third medication check, verifying the patient identification and the correct time.
8. Verify the patient's allergies and that there is no allergy to the piggyback medication.
9. Assess for side effects of a previous dose of the same medication. If adverse effects have occurred, withhold the medication and notify the physician.
10. Hang the minibag (piggyback) medication on the other arm of the IV pole.
11. Lower the main IV container using the hanger that came with the secondary tubing set.
12. Cleanse the lowest Y-site injection port on the administration set tubing.
13. Attach the secondary tubing to the Y-site injection port.
14. Open the roller clamp on the secondary set and regulate the flow to the desired rate.
15. Chart the medication.
16. Return when the time for the piggyback medication to infuse has ended.
17. Remove the secondary set and empty the piggyback container.
18. Raise the primary IV container and re-regulate the flow to the ordered rate.
19. Discard the empty piggyback container appropriately.
20. Note the amount of the piggyback medication that infused on the I&O sheet.

Guidelines for Monitoring a Blood Transfusion

Students are not allowed to administer blood products, but are often asked to monitor the patient who is receiving a blood transfusion. The student should accompany the nurse through each step of the process to become familiar with the procedure and safeguards used when administering blood products.

Nursing Considerations

▼ Double-check the physician's order.

▼ Verify that a consent for blood administration has been signed.

▼ Assess to determine if the patient has ever had a transfusion reaction.

▼ Administer any medications ordered to prevent transfusion reaction (e.g., antipyretic, antihistamine, or steroid).

▼ Verify that the correct size of IV cannula is in place (an 18-gauge cannula is preferable; a 20-gauge may be used for some blood products).

▼ Use a Y-type blood administration set of tubing with filter. The blood container is attached to one side of the Y and a container of normal saline is attached to the other side of the Y.

▼ **Before the container of blood is attached to the patient, the label is checked with the blood bracelet and ID band on the patient by two nurses**. Two identifiers are used such as patient name and hospital ID number. This is to verify the correct patient, blood type, and correct unit match the patient's blood. The numbers must match between the blood container and the blood band on the patient's arm. The ID check should include the following:
  - The patient's full name (check armband and ask the patient)
  - Patient's hospital number
  - Blood unit number
  - Blood group, Rh factor, and ABO designation
  - Expiration date
  - Type and cross-match number

▼ Baseline vital signs, including temperature, are taken just before the blood transfusion is started.

▼ Use only saline (0.9% NaCl) before or during the transfusion in the same IV tubing. Start the saline, slowly, before the blood arrives from the blood bank.

▼ Blood infusions must be started within 30 minutes of arrival on the unit; otherwise, return the blood to the blood bank. Blood may not be stored in the unit refrigerator.

▼ Stay with the patient for the first 15 minutes of the infusion. Monitor closely for signs of complications.

▼ Complications that may occur during infusion include high fever, sudden chills, headache, flushing, tachycardia, hypotension, itching, hives, rash, wheezing, shortness of breath, lower back pain, distention of neck veins, oppressive feeling in chest, sense of impending doom. Should any of these symptoms occur, stop the infusion, start saline to run slowly, stay with the patient, and notify another nurse to call the physician. (The student also should notify the instructor.)

▼ Vital signs are taken after 15 minutes and then every half hour until the infusion is complete.

▼ **Do not allow blood to hang for more than 4 hours.**

▼ If a reaction occurs, return the unit of blood to the blood bank with the appropriate information concerning the reaction.

▼ Monitor the patient closely for an additional hour after the transfusion. Continue to monitor during the following days for delayed reactions, such as hematuria (blood in the urine).

ACID-BASE IMBALANCES

Respiratory Acidosis			Respiratory Alkalosis		
Causes: Carbonic acid excess usually resulting from respiratory compromise/failure			**Causes:** Carbonic acid deficit usually resulting from hyperventilation (natural or mechanical)		
	Uncompensated	*Compensated*		*Uncompensated*	*Compensated*
pH	<7.35	↑	pH	>7.35	Normal
pCO₂	↑	↑	pCO₂	↑	↑
HCO₃	Normal	↑	HCO₃	Normal	↑
Metabolic Acidosis			**Metabolic Alkalosis**		
Causes: Bicarbonate deficit due to renal failure, starvation, high-protein diet.			**Causes:** Bicarbonate excess due to hyperkalemia, excessive vomiting, diuretic therapy, etc.		
	Uncompensated	*Compensated*		*Uncompensated*	*Compensated*
pH	<7.35	Normal	pH	>7.35	Normal
pCO₂	Normal	↓	pCO₂	Normal	↑
HCO₃	↓	↓	HCO₃	↑	↑

Adapted from *Mosby's Nursing PDQ for LPN,* St Louis, 2005, Elsevier, p 55.

CLINICAL GUIDELINES
Guide to Standard References

▼ *Physicians' Desk Reference* (PDR)—Contains information on drugs organized by generic drug name, brand name, or category of use. This book is available on most nursing units. Use it to find pertinent information about drugs you will be giving.

▼ *Procedure Manual*—A thick book containing the accepted procedure for performing various nursing skills in the clinical facility. This book is an in-house volume and may vary in content from one clinical facility to another. Use it to review each nursing procedure before preparing to do it (e.g., urinary catheterization, sterile dressing change).

▼ *Diet Manual*—A listing of foods allowed and forbidden on the various therapeutic diets available in the clinical facility. Use this manual to check what the patient may and may not have when a special diet is prescribed.

▼ *Documentation/Charting Manual*—A manual designating the accepted procedures and forms to be used for documentation of nursing care within the particular clinical facility. Use this manual to learn to document correctly the nursing care you give.

▼ *Medical Dictionary*—Provides definitions of medical terms, pronunciations of words, correct spelling of medical words, lists of abbreviations, and a variety of appendices that may include lists of symbols, prefixes and suffixes, nursing diagnoses, diagnosis-related groups (DRGs), tables of laboratory values, foreign language terms, anatomic tables or charts, food value charts, and other helpful aids.

▼ *Clinical Nursing Manual*—A Manual of Nursing Practice, Manual of Nursing Therapeutics, Manual of Clinical Nursing, or books with similar titles that contain information about most procedures and client conditions generally encountered by the average staff nurse.

Preparing the Preoperative Patient

▼ Check that the surgical consent has been signed.

▼ Check if a blood permit was required and that it was signed.

▼ Verify that the complete blood count, urinalysis, and other required diagnostic test data are on the chart.

▼ Bathe or shower the patient and dress in clean gown only (no underwear).

▼ Check that preoperative medications are available on the unit.

▼ Calculate any preoperative medication dosages that will be needed.

▼ Remove jewelry and place all valuables in valuables envelope for safekeeping, or give them to a family member. (A wedding band may be tied or taped in place.)

▼ Check and inquire about any piercings with body jewelry any place on the body. If metal jewelry is left in place, the patient may be burned from the electrical cautery used during surgery. Remove the jewelry.

▼ Remove all metal pins from hair.

▼ Prepare the preoperative checklist form that accompanies the patient to surgery.

▼ One-half hour before the patient is expected to go to surgery, have him or her empty the bladder and remove dentures (if required).

▼ Prepare and administer any/ordered preoperative medication at the time it is scheduled to be taken, with the supervision of the instructor or nurse as required.

▼ Lower the bed, raise the side rails, place call light within reach, and caution the patient not to get up.

▼ Finish charting in nurse's notes.

▼ The area to be operated on (for example, the right knee) is marked with indelible ink before the surgical procedure with the patient's verification, either in the patient's room or in the holding room in the surgical suite; follow agency protocol. This is best done before preoperative medication is administered.

▼ When the transporter comes to take the patient to surgery, the patient is correlated with the transport slip, using two patient identifiers on the chart and patient ID band. Usually name and hospital ID number are used. The chart and the patient are correlated in the same manner.

Care and Assessment of the Postoperative Patient on Return to the Clinical Unit

▼ Obtain report from the recovery room nurse who cared for the patient in the postanesthesia care unit (PACU).

▼ Note time of return to the unit and quickly scan the postoperative orders.

▼ Transfer to bed and provide warmth.

▼ Take vital signs and compare with previous data.

▼ Assess wound and dressing; check drains; note amount and type of drainage; check or connect/compress wound suction devices.

▼ Position for safety and comfort (usually on side with head up 15 to 30 degrees).

▼ Assess color and temperature of skin.

▼ Assess area/system involved in the surgery (e.g., check abdominal girth, distal pulses, movement of body parts, and so forth).

▼ Check length of each tube for patency and function: urinary catheter, IV lines, chest tubes, oxygen cannula, and the like. Attach to drainage device or suction as ordered.

▼ Check intravenous infusion for correct solution, additives, and rate of flow; assess site.

▼ Assess urinary status: time of last voiding, amount of fluids infused, bladder distention, urge to void, amount of hourly output via catheter. *(Do not infuse intravenous fluid containing potassium until urine output is at least 30 mL/hr.)*

▼ Assess neurologic status: level of consciousness, orientation, ease of arousal, ability to move extremities.

▼ Assess pain: verbal complaint, body language, time of previous analgesia, if any; medicate as needed per orders.

▼ Assess for nausea: medicate as needed per orders.

▼ Attach call light and place emesis basin and tissues within reach.

▼ Assure patient that the surgery is over and that he or she is safely back in the nursing unit.

▼ Allow family members to see patient briefly.

Blood Pressure Parameters and Classification

Classification	Systolic Measurement		Diastolic Measurement
Normal	<120	and	<80
Prehypertension	120-139	or	80-89
Stage I hypertension	140-159	or	90-99
Stage II hypertension	≥160	or	≥100

Glasgow Coma Scale

This scale is used to assess the condition of patients who have a decreased level of consciousness or who are at risk for a decreasing level of consciousness or neurologic injury. Assess each category of response and add up the score.

Category of Response	Stimulus	Response	Score
Eye opening	Approach to bedside	Spontaneous response	4
	Verbal command	Opening of eyes to name or command	3
	Pain	Opening of eye only to pain	2
		Lack of eye opening to any stimulus	1
Best verbal response	Verbal questioning with maximum arousal	Appropriate orientation, conversant, correct identification of self, year, month, and place	5
		Confusion, disorientation in one or more areas, but is conversant	4
		Inappropriate use of words, cursing, lack of sustained conversation	3
		Incomprehensible words, moaning	2
		Lack of sound with any stimuli	1
Best motor response	Verbal command	Obedience to the command	6
	Pain (pressure on proximal nailbed)	Lack of obedience but attempts to remove offending stimulus	5
		Flexion withdrawl*	4
		Abnormal flexion, flexing of arm at elbow and pronation, making a fist	3
		Abnormal extension, extension of arm at elbow with adduction and internal rotation of arm at shoulder	2
		Lack of response	1

The highest possible score is 15. The higher the score, the better the condition of the patient.

*For example, "Raise your arm, hold up two fingers."
Adapted from Lewis SM, Heitkemper MM, Dirksen SR, O'Brien PG, Bucher L: *Medical-surgical nursing: assessment and management of clinical problems*, ed 7, St Louis, 2007, Mosby, p 1477.

POSTOPERATIVE EXERCISES TO PREVENT COMPLICATIONS
Deep Breathing and Coughing

▼ Place patient in a sitting position, preferably on the side of the bed so that lung expansion is not restricted by the mattress. May use semi-Fowler's or side position with the head of the bed elevated 30 to 40 degrees.

▼ If the patient has a thoracic or an abdominal incision, splint the area with a small pillow or tightly folded towel; show the patient how to do this. Hold the splinting material tightly over the incision.

▼ Ask the patient to inhale as deeply as possible through the nose, hold the breath for a count of five, and then slowly exhale completely through the mouth. Repeat four to six times.

▼ On the last deep breath, ask the patient to cough forcibly on exhalation. If unable to perform a full cough, ask the patient to exhale forcibly with the mouth open several times in a row to "huff" cough and move secretions up the bronchial tree so that they can be expectorated.

▼ Repeat deep breathing and coughing at least every 2 hours, and ask patient to deep breathe every hour, or whenever a commercial comes on the TV, or a page of reading material is turned. *This is the most effective way to prevent postoperative respiratory complications.*

Using the Incentive Spirometer Correctly

Instruct the patient to do the following:

▼ Place the mouthpiece in mouth and completely cover it with the lips.

▼ Take a slow, deep breath and hold it for at least 3 seconds.

▼ Exhale slowly, with the lips puckered.

▼ Breathe normally for a few breaths.

▼ Increase the inspired volume, if possible, by 100 mL with each breath.

▼ When maximal volume is attained, attempt to reach it 10 times, resting a few breaths in between each attempt.

Leg Exercises

▼ Ask the patient to flex each foot firmly, pointing the toes toward the ceiling, and then to extend the foot fully and firmly. This contracts and relaxes the calf and thigh muscles (gastrocnemius and quadriceps). Repeat five times.

▼ Ask the patient to rotate the ankles so that the toes draw circles, first in one direction and then the other. Repeat five times.

▼ Ask the patient to raise and lower the legs by bending and flexing at the knee. Repeat five times. If the patient has an abdominal incision, raise the head of the bed 30 to 40 degrees before doing this exercise to relieve pressure on the abdominal muscles.

▼ Ask the patient to press the back of the knee against the mattress and then relax it if quadriceps setting exercises are ordered. Repeat 10 to 12 times an hour.

Turning in Bed and Ambulation

▼ Assist the patient to turn in bed at least every 2 hours (preferably every hour) in a side-to-back-to-side pattern as permitted. Position in proper body alignment, providing pillow support to the back, leg joints, and arms as needed.

▼ Prepare the patient by having him or her turn to the side and then push up to a sitting position, or raise the head of the bed with the patient supine and then pivot the legs and upper body so that he or she is sitting on the side of the bed.

▼ Allow the patient to sit on the side of the bed with the feet supported either on the floor or on a stool. (Place slippers on the feet.) Allow several minutes of sitting the first time up after surgery. Otherwise, a couple of minutes should be sufficient before rising to a standing position.

▼ Assist the patient to a standing position and allow time for stabilization of blood pressure before beginning ambulation. Support the patient appropriately.

▼ Assist with ambulation by providing the needed amount of support and assistance. Ambulate half the total distance planned because the patient will need to return to bed or the chair.

▼ Rubber-soled slippers are safest for ambulation. Provide warmth with a robe or other cover as needed. Remember to remove the robe before placing the patient back on the bed.

PAIN ASSESSMENT
JCAHO Pain Standards

The following is a summary of the standards for pain assessment for all patients in any setting from the Joint Commission on Accreditation of Healthcare Organizations (JCAHO):

1. Patients have the right to appropriate assessment and management of pain.
2. Pain will be assessed in all patients in a timely and recurring manner.
3. Policies and procedures must support safe medication prescription or ordering.
4. Patients must be educated about pain and managing pain as part of treatment, as appropriate.
5. The discharge process will provide for continuing pain care based on the patient's assessed needs at the time of discharge.
6. Organizations will collect data to monitor their performance, addressing the following areas:
   ▼ Appropriate pain assessment and management
   ▼ Effective pain treatment or referral for treatment
   ▼ Timely assessment and reassessment of pain, including the nature and intensity
   ▼ Patient involvement in making decisions about pain management
   ▼ Education for staff and patients regarding the following:
      a. The importance of effective pain management
      b. Pain management as a part of total treatment

   c. Continuing pain care after discharge

   d. Documentation of pain assessments, treatments, and evaluation of effectiveness

   e. Staff competency in pain assessment and management

Pain is considered the "fifth vital sign" and should be assessed whenever vital signs are taken.

   After assessment, documentation of the findings must be completed. Numerous pain assessment tools are available. Use the scale that is designated in the pain assessment procedure for your agency.

Pain Scales

Numerical Pain Scale. Rate your pain on a scale of 1 to 10, with 1 being almost no pain and 10 being unbearable pain.

Wong-Baker FACES Pain Rating Scale (Figure 5-7)

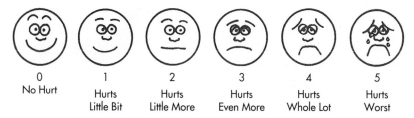

Wong-Baker FACES Pain Rating Scale

0	1	2	3	4	5
No Hurt	Hurts Little Bit	Hurts Little More	Hurts Even More	Hurts Whole Lot	Hurts Worst

FIGURE 5-7 *Brief word instructions:* Point to each face using the words to describe the pain intensity. Ask the person to choose the face that best describes his or her own pain and record the appropriate number. *Original instructions:* Explain to the person that each face is for a person who feels happy because he has no pain (hurt) or sad because he has some or a lot of pain. Face 0 is very happy because he doesn't hurt at all. Face 1 hurts just a little bit. Face 2 hurts a little more. Face 3 hurts even more. Face 4 hurts a whole lot. Face 5 hurts as much as you can imagine, although you don't have to be crying to feel this bad. Ask the person to choose the face that best describes how he or she is feeling. Rating scale is recommended for persons ages 3 years and older. (From Hockenberry MJ: *Wong's essentials of pediatric nursing*, ed 7, St Louis, 2005, Mosby, p 1259.)

Descriptive Word Rating Scale. Chart rating over scale (e.g., 3/5).

0	1	2	3	4	5
No pain	Mild	Discomforting	Distressing	Horrible	Excruciating

Visual Analogue Scale (VAS). Have the patient indicate the degree of pain by marking the line below:

   *No pain at all*_____*Greatest pain possible*

Verbal Descriptor Scale (VDS). Have the patient check the best descriptor of his or her pain at this moment (may read to the resident):

__ absent	__ severe
__ minimal	__ very severe
__ mild	__ extremely severe
__ moderate	__ exquisite
__ fairly severe	__ unbearable

FLACC Scale

	0	1	2
Face	No particular expression or smile	Occasional grimace or frown, withdrawn, disinterested	Frequent to constant frown, clenched jaw, quivering chin
Legs	Normal position or relaxed	Uneasy, restless, tense	Kicking, or legs drawn up
Activity	Lying quietly, normal position, moves easily	Squirming, shifting back and forth, tense	Arched, rigid, or jerking
Cry	No cry (awake or asleep)	Moans or whimpers, occasional complaint	Crying steadily, screams or sobs, frequent complaints
Consolability	Content, relaxed	Reassured by occasional touching, hugging, or talking to, distractible	Difficult to console or comfort

The FLACC is a behavior pain assessment scale created by the University of Michigan Medical Center (can be reproduced for clinical and research use). It's useful for pain assessment in the elderly, confused, or noncommunicative patient.

Memory Device for Assessment of Chest Pain: PQRST

Factor	Questions to Ask
P—Precipitating events	What events or factors precipitated the pain or discomfort (e.g., activity, exercise, resting)?
Q—Quality of pain or discomfort	What does the pain or discomfort feel like (e.g., dull, aching, sharp, tight)?

Continued

Memory Device for Assessment of Chest Pain: PQRST—cont'd

Factor	Questions to Ask
R—Radiation of pain	Where is the pain located? Where does the pain radiate to (e.g., back, arms, jaw, teeth, shoulder, elbow)?
S—Severity of pain	On a scale of 0 to 10 with 10 being the most severe pain, how would you rate the pain or discomfort?
T—Timing	When did the pain or discomfort begin? Has the pain changed since that time? Have you had pain like this before?

This memory device may be used for pain in other locations as well.

From Lewis SM, Heitkemper MM, Dirksen SR, O'Brien PG, Bucher L: *Medical-surgical nursing: assessment and management of clinical problems,* ed 7, St Louis, 2007, Mosby.

Measures to Relieve Pain and Discomfort

▼ Relieve extraneous sensory input by providing a quiet, tidy environment.
▼ Administer pain medication promptly; assess patient for pain level at the time the next dose could be given.
▼ Advise patient to ask for pain medication before pain becomes severe; medication is more effective if given before the onset of severe pain.
▼ Provide distraction with reading material, a TV program, pleasant music, or conversation.
▼ Offer a massage.
▼ Teach relaxation exercises.
▼ Assist with a pleasant imagery exercise.
▼ Straighten bed linens and position for comfort.
▼ Seek to reduce anxieties if possible.
▼ Encourage verbalization of fears.
▼ Provide other analgesic between narcotic doses, if ordered.
▼ Encourage use of heat or cold treatments as ordered.
▼ Determine if pain medication ordered is effective; if not, request an order change from the physician.
▼ Remember that just because a patient may go to sleep, it does not mean that the pain medication is not needed.

Equianalgesic Doses of Opioids

Drug	Equianalgesic Dose*	
	Parenteral	Oral
Agents for Mild to Moderate Pain		
Codeine†	130 mg q3-4h	200 mg q3-4h
Hydrocodone	NA	30 mg q3-4h
Oxycodone	NA	15 mg q3-4h
Oxycodone SR	NA	45-60 mg q12h

Equianalgesic Doses of Opioids—cont'd

	Equianalgesic Dose*	
Drug	Parenteral	Oral
Agents for Moderate to Severe Pain		
Morphine	10 mg q3-4h	30 mg q3-4h
Morphine SR	NA	90-120 mg q12h
Morphine ER	NA	180-240 mg q24h
Hydromorphone	1.5 mg q3-4h	7.5 mg q3-4h
Levorphanol	2 mg q6-8h	4 mg q6-8h
Methadone	1 mg q6-8h	20 mg q6-8h
Oxymorphone	1 mg q3-4h	NA
Fentanyl	100 mcg/h (subcut., IV, or transdermal)	
	equals 4 mg/hr IV morphine	

SR, Sustained release; *ER*, extended release; *NA*, not available.
*Equianalgesic dose = dose that will produce the same degree of analgesia as 10 mg of parenteral morphine given every 3 to 4 hours.
†Codeine is not generally recommended for chronic therapy because the doses required to produce significant analgesia also produce significant side effects.
From Lehne RA: *Pharmacology for nursing care,* ed 5, Philadelphia, 2004, Saunders.

FALL RISK FACTORS

The risk of falling becomes greater when a patient becomes ill. Fever, electrolyte imbalance, and dulled mental alertness often contribute to a fall. This is especially true for the elderly patient. General factors that contribute to falls include the following:

▼ Medications that cause postural hypotension or dizziness; polypharmacy (sedatives, hypnotics, antihypertensives, diuretics, antidepressants, laxatives)
▼ Muscle weakness from inactivity or illness
▼ Neuropathy in the feet and legs (diabetes)
▼ Vision problems or dirty glasses
▼ Balance or gait problem (poststroke or neurologic disorder)
▼ Alcohol use
▼ Mental changes; dementia, delirium
▼ Incontinence and urgency
▼ Neurologic diseases (stroke, Parkinson's disease, multiple sclerosis, etc.)
▼ Illness and fever
▼ Severe osteoporosis and spontaneous fracture
▼ Environmental hazards (scatter rugs, pets, stairs, slippery floors or showers, small objects on floors, cords in pathways)

Often it is a combination of factors that causes a person to fall.

SCALE OF PITTING EDEMA

To assess for pitting edema, depress the skin with your fingertips over the tibia or the medial malleolus for 5 seconds and then release.

Normally there is no edema except during pregnancy or when the person has been standing all day.

1+ = Trace	Pit is barely seen 2 mm depth
2+ = Mild	Pit is deeper and rebounds within a few seconds 4 mm depth
3+ = Moderate	Deep pit is formed 6 mm depth
4+ = Severe	Deeper pit is formed that may take more than 30 seconds to rebound 8 mm depth

From Christensen BL, Kockrow EO: *Foundations of nursing*, ed 4, St Louis, 2002, Mosby.

ASSESSMENT OF SKIN PRESSURE POINTS

Pressure points (Figure 5-8) should be examined whenever a patient is repositioned, but must be assessed every 2 hours for the immobilized patient.

Factors That Contribute to Pressure Ulcer Risk

Consider patients with the following problems as having high risk for skin breakdown and pressure ulcers:
▼ Immobility (stroke, paraplegia, quadriplegia)
▼ Malnutrition and low body weight; hypoalbuminemia
▼ Dehydration
▼ Incontinence
▼ Anemia
▼ Peripheral vascular disease
▼ Diabetes mellitus
▼ Dementia
▼ Edema
▼ Dry skin
▼ Fractures
▼ Malignancy
▼ Infection

Staging for Pressure Ulcers

The following staging criteria are recommended by the National Pressure Ulcer Advisory Panel and the Agency for Health Care Policy and Research (AHCPR). Pressure ulcers, once originally staged, should

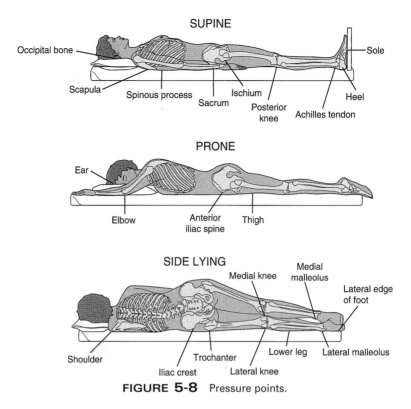

FIGURE 5-8 Pressure points.

not be "reverse staged"—that is, a stage IV ulcer remains a stage IV until it becomes a "healed stage IV." Healing is documented by improvement in wound size, depth, amount of necrotic tissue, and amount of exudate. Eschar must be debrided before proper staging can occur.

Stage I: Pressure alteration of skin as compared to adjacent area such as change in skin temperature (warmness or coolness), tissue consistency (firm or boggy feel), and/or sensation (pain, itching). A defined area of persistent redness in lightly pigmented skin, or in darker skin tones, an area of persistent red, blue, or purple hues. Discoloration does not blanch with fingertip pressure.

Stage II: Partial-thickness skin loss involving epidermis, dermis, or both. May appear as an abrasion, a blister, or a shallow crater. Area around damaged skin may feel warm.

Stage III: Full-thickness skin loss involving damage to, or necrosis of, subcutaneous tissue that may extend down to, but not through, underlying fascia. A deep crater with or without undermining of adjacent tissue. Bacterial infection with drainage may be present. Surrounding tissue may be damaged.

Stage IV: Full-thickness skin loss with extensive destruction, tissue necrosis, or damage to muscle, bone, or supporting structures (e.g., tendon, joint capsule). Undermining and sinus tracts (tunnels) also may be associated with stage IV pressure ulcers. Infection is often present. May appear dry and black, with a buildup of tough, necrotic tissue (eschar), or it can appear wet and oozing.

GUIDELINES FOR CAST CARE

▼ Check the cast for integrity: no breaks, cracks, crumbling edges.
▼ Assess the degree of tightness around the casted part: it should not be cutting into the flesh.
▼ **Assess for circulation and movement distal to the cast: check pulses, skin temperature, ability to move joints, and sensation.**
▼ Assess for any pain related to the placement of the cast.
▼ Feel along the cast for "hot" spots that might indicate underlying infection.
▼ Smell the ends of the cast for any odor, indicating the presence of infection.
▼ Position the casted area per the physician's orders; support joints proximal and distal to the cast.
▼ Supervise range-of-motion exercises for joints proximal or distal to the cast as ordered.
▼ Caution patient not to poke anything under the cast.
▼ Handle a cast that is still wet with the flat of the palm of the hand rather than the fingertips when positioning.
▼ Listen to what the patient says, and heed any complaints with further exploration of the problem.

GUIDELINES FOR TRACTION CARE

▼ Check the physician's order regarding the type of traction and amount of weight to be used.
▼ Assess the traction setup and verify the following:
  ▪ Weights are hanging free.
  ▪ Patient's body is in correct alignment.
  ▪ Traction components are positioned and functioning properly.
▼ Perform pin care as ordered if pins are in place.
▼ Make the bed from top to bottom, rather than side to side, with an assistant.
▼ Keep linens smooth under the patient.
▼ Obtain a trapeze bar so the patient can assist with repositioning.
▼ Assess the area of injury for signs of infection; check for "hot" areas, drainage, and foul smell.
▼ Assess the need for pain medication on a regular schedule.
▼ Assess for systemic signs of infection (e.g., elevated white blood cell count, elevated temperature, increasing malaise).
▼ Offer bed pan frequently or on a set schedule per patient's elimination pattern.
▼ Track frequency of bowel movements and take action if none occur for 3 days.
▼ Supervise range-of-motion exercises for other joints, especially in older patients.

SUBSTANCE ABUSE SCREENING QUESTIONS: CAGE

C **Cut down:** "Have you ever felt you ought to **cut down** on your drinking or drug use?"

A **Annoyed:** "Have people **annoyed** you by criticizing your drinking or drug use?"

G **Guilty:** "Have you felt bad or **guilty** about your drinking or drug use?"

E **Eye-opener:** "Have you ever had a drink or used drugs first thing in the morning to steady your nerves or get rid of a hangover **(eye-opener)**?"

The answer "yes" to any of the above questions indicates that the patient may have a substance abuse problem.

Adapted from *Mosby's nursing PDQ for LPN,* St Louis, 2005, Mosby.

MEASURES TO ASSIST THE PATIENT TO URINATE

With the patient positioned for urination:

▽ Run water in a nearby sink.

▽ Have the female patient blow through a straw into a glass of water.

▽ Assist a male patient to stand at the bedside (with a physician's order).

▽ Allow privacy if patient can be left alone.

▽ Gently, but firmly, use Credé movements over the bladder (massage from top of bladder to bottom by rocking the palm of the hand over it).

▽ Place patient in a warm sitz bath (with physician's order). Encourage to void into the sitz bath. Cleanse perineum afterward.

▽ Pour warm water over the perineum with patient attempting to void. Place the patient's hand in a bowl or pan of warm water.

▽ Encourage patient to breathe deep and relax; ask patient to visualize running water in a peaceful place.

MEASURES TO RELIEVE FLATULENCE (GAS)

▽ Ambulate in an upright position as much as possible.

▽ Seek an order for simethicone medication to decrease gas formation.

▽ Avoid carbonated beverages, beverages containing ice, and gas-forming foods.

▽ Avoid drinking through a straw (it increases the swallowing of air, which causes gas).

▽ Use abdominal massage if not contraindicated; massage with a circular motion over the large intestine, moving in the direction that intestinal contents travel. This encourages gas to move down the intestinal tract.

▽ Use measures to stimulate a bowel movement, such as warm water with lemon juice, a rectal suppository (if ordered), or measures that usually work for the particular patient.

▽ Obtain an order for the insertion of a rectal tube.

▼ If discomfort is severe, ask the physician if the patient can be placed in Trendelenburg position for short periods of time to encourage gas to move out of the intestine. (With the intestine and rectum higher than the stomach and head, the gas will move up and out.)

NUTRITIONAL CARE
A Guide to Daily Food Choices

Use MyPyramid (Figure 5-9) to help you eat better every day — the Dietary Guidelines way. Note the 2005 Dietary Guidelines on the next page:

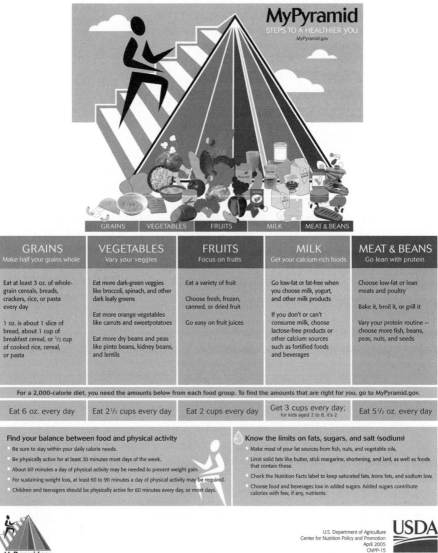

GRAINS	VEGETABLES	FRUITS	MILK	MEAT & BEANS
Make half your grains whole	Vary your veggies	Focus on fruits	Get your calcium-rich foods	Go lean with protein
Eat at least 3 oz. of whole-grain cereals, breads, crackers, rice, or pasta every day	Eat more dark-green veggies like broccoli, spinach, and other dark leafy greens	Eat a variety of fruit	Go low-fat or fat-free when you choose milk, yogurt, and other milk products	Choose low-fat or lean meats and poultry
		Choose fresh, frozen, canned, or dried fruit		Bake it, broil it, or grill it
1 oz. is about 1 slice of bread, about 1 cup of breakfast cereal, or ½ cup of cooked rice, cereal, or pasta	Eat more orange vegetables like carrots and sweetpotatoes	Go easy on fruit juices	If you don't or can't consume milk, choose lactose-free products or other calcium sources such as fortified foods and beverages	Vary your protein routine — choose more fish, beans, peas, nuts, and seeds
	Eat more dry beans and peas like pinto beans, kidney beans, and lentils			

For a 2,000-calorie diet, you need the amounts below from each food group. To find the amounts that are right for you, go to MyPyramid.gov.

| Eat 6 oz. every day | Eat 2½ cups every day | Eat 2 cups every day | Get 3 cups every day; for kids aged 2 to 8, it's 2 | Eat 5½ oz. every day |

Find your balance between food and physical activity
- Be sure to stay within your daily calorie needs.
- Be physically active for at least 30 minutes most days of the week.
- About 60 minutes a day of physical activity may be needed to prevent weight gain.
- For sustaining weight loss, at least 60 to 90 minutes a day of physical activity may be required.
- Children and teenagers should be physically active for 60 minutes every day, or most days.

Know the limits on fats, sugars, and salt (sodium)
- Make most of your fat sources from fish, nuts, and vegetable oils.
- Limit solid fats like butter, stick margarine, shortening, and lard, as well as foods that contain these.
- Check the Nutrition Facts label to keep saturated fats, trans fats, and sodium low.
- Choose food and beverages low in added sugars. Added sugars contribute calories with few, if any, nutrients.

MyPyramid.gov
STEPS TO A HEALTHIER YOU

U.S. Department of Agriculture
Center for Nutrition Policy and Promotion
April 2005
CNPP-15

USDA is an equal opportunity provider and employer

FIGURE 5-9   MyPyramid. (From U.S. Department of Health and Human Services/U.S. Department of Agriculture, 2005.)

▼ Fruits and vegetables: Consume 2 cups of fruit and 2½ cups of vegetables daily. Make fruits and vegetables half of what is eaten at each meal. Choose fiber-rich fruits and vegetables.

▼ Whole grains: 6 ounces. Eat three 1-ounce portions of whole grains. Choose whole, unsweetened grains when possible.

▼ Dairy products: Drink 3 cups of skim or low-fat milk or eat the equivalent dairy products: low-fat yogurt or low-fat cheese.

▼ Protein: Eat 5½ ounces of poultry, lean meat, fish, beans, or nuts. Eat meat rarely. Choose lean meats and poultry. Bake, broil, or grill meat, poultry, and fish choices.

▼ Oils and sweets: 6 teaspoons per day used sparingly. Use healthful oils such as olive, canola, and safflower. Sugar should be limited. Keep total fat intake between 20% and 35% of calories, with most fats coming from sources of polysaturated and monounsaturated fatty acids, such as fish, nuts, and vegetable oils. Consume less than 10% of calories from saturated fatty acids and less than 300 mg/day of cholesterol, and keep trans fatty acid consumption as low as possible.

Calorie control is to be considered as well for a healthy diet. Combine a healthy diet with sufficient exercise to maintain a healthy weight.

Choice Equivalents within Each Food Group

The guidelines are based on a 2000-calorie diet.

What is a serving?

Fruits: 2 cups of fruit a day. Eat a variety and use fresh, frozen, canned, or dried fruit rather than fruit juice. A serving could be 1 small banana, 1 medium orange, or ¼ cup of dried apricots or peaches.

Vegetables: 2½ cups a day. In particular, select from all five vegetable subgroups (dark green, orange, legumes, starchy vegetables, and other vegetables) several times a week. Eat portions of vegetables for lunch and dinner.

Grains: 6 ounces per day. 3 ounce equivalents a day of whole-grain products. Half the grains should be whole grains. One ounce is 1 slice of bread, 1 cup of breakfast cereal, or ½ cup of cooked rice or pasta.

Protein: 5½ ounces of poultry, lean meat, fish, beans, or nuts per day. Equivalent servings of 1 ounce of meat, fish, or poultry are as follows: 1 egg, ¼ cup cooked beans, 1 tablespoon of peanut butter, ½ ounce of nuts or seeds, and ¼ cup of tofu. A 4-ounce serving of meat, fish, or poultry for dinner should be about the size of a normal deck of cards, or about the size of the palm of the hand.

Dairy products: 3 cups of milk per day. 1 cup of milk equals 8 ounces. Equivalent servings to 1 cup of milk are 1 cup of low-fat or nonfat yogurt, ½ ounce of low-fat cheese such as Swiss, Gouda, Roquefort, or white string cheese. 2 ounces of low-fat or fat-free processed cheese such as American or Laughing Cow is equal to 1 cup of milk.

Fats: 6 teaspoons per day. 1 teaspoon of liquid oil is equal to 1 teaspoon of tub margarine, 1 tablespoon of mayonnaise, or 2 teaspoons of light salad dressing.

Major Key Recommendations

Balance body weight in a healthy range; balance calories from foods and beverages with calories expended.

Those who choose to drink alcoholic beverages should do so sensibly and in moderation—defined as the consumption of up to one drink per day for women and up to two drinks per day for men.

Consume less than 2300 mg (approximately 1 tsp of salt) of sodium per day. Choose and prepare foods with little salt. At the same time, consume potassium-rich foods, such as fruits and vegetables.

Children and adolescents. Children 2 to 8 years of age should consume 2 cups per day of fat-free or low-fat milk or equivalent milk products. Children 9 years of age and older should consume 3 cups per day of fat-free or low-fat milk or equivalent milk products.

Women of childbearing age who may become pregnant. Eat iron-rich plant foods or iron-fortified foods along with vitamin C–rich foods. Consume adequate folate foods daily or adequate synthetic folic acid from a supplement.

Women in the first trimester of pregnancy. Consume adequate synthetic folic acid daily from fortified foods or supplements in addition to folate food forms.

People over age 50. Consume vitamin B_{12} in its crystalline form (i.e., fortified foods or supplements).

Older adults, people with dark skin, and people exposed to insufficient ultraviolet sunlight. Consume extra vitamin D from vitamin D–fortified foods and/or supplements.

All populations. Engage in regular physical activity and reduce sedentary activities to promote health, psychologic well-being, and a healthy body weight.

Body Mass Index

The body mass index (BMI) is based on the relationship of weight to height. It is independent of body frame size. BMI is used to determine if the person has excess fat. Body mass is calculated with the following formula:

$$BMI = \frac{Weight\ (lb)}{Height\ (in)^2} \times 705$$

In the adult, a score of 20 to 25 is associated with the least risk of early death.

Example: A woman 5 ft 4 in tall, weighing 122 lb
Height squared = 64 in × 64 in = 4096
122 ÷ 4096 = 0.0297085
0.029785 × 705 = 20.9

This woman's body mass index is 20.9.

Therapeutic Diets

Clear Liquid Diet

Purpose: Provides an oral source of calories and electrolytes as a means of preventing dehydration and reducing colonic residue to a minimum.

Indications: The immediate postoperative period, acute debilitation, acute gastroenteritis, upper gastrointestinal lesions; also to reduce the amount of residue in the colon in preparation for bowel surgery, barium enema, or after colon surgery.

Type of Food	Foods Included	Foods Excluded
Beverage	Carbonated beverages, tea, coffee, strained fruit juice (apple, cranberry, cranapple, grape, punch, powdered fruit beverage mixes, electrolyte replacement drinks)	Milk, milk drinks
Soup	Fat-free bouillon or broth, consommé	Any other
Dessert	Plain gelatin, Popsicles, fruit ice	Any other
Condiments	Sugar, honey, plain hard candy No caffeine, no artificial sweetner	Any other

Full Liquid Diet

Indications: Oral surgery, mandibular fracture, plastic surgery to the face, esophageal strictures; also for acutely ill client for whom chewing may be difficult, or other postoperative states in transition between a clear liquid and other diet; three to six small feedings a day are recommended.

Contraindications: Nausea, vomiting, distention, or diarrhea when advanced to this diet postoperatively, lactose intolerance.

Type of Food	Foods Included	Foods Excluded
Beverage	Carbonated beverages, coffee, tea, fruit juices, milk, milk drinks, vegetable juices (strained), eggnog	None
Bread	None	All
Cereal	Soft-cooked cereals (gruels)	Any other
Fat	Butter, cream, margarine	Any other
Vegetables	Tomato juice, vegetable puree in soup	Any other
Meat, egg, cheese	Raw pasteurized eggs.* Soft-cooked egg sometimes allowed	Any other
Soup	Broth, strained cream soups, yogurt	Any other
Dessert	Yogurt, custard, ice cream (plain), pudding, tapioca, sherbets, plain gelatin	Any other
Condiments	Pepper, salt, cinnamon, nutmeg, sugar, honey, hard candy, syrup, pureed meat and vegetables for soup only	Any other

*Raw, unpasteurized eggs should not be used because of the danger of *Salmonella* infection. In addition, the avidin in the egg white prevents the absorption of biotin.

Adapted from Pekenpaugh N, Poleman C: *Nutrition: essentials and diet therapy*, ed 10, Philadelphia, 2007, Saunders, pp 482-483. Reprinted with permission.

Soft, Low-Fiber Diet

Indications: Gastrointestinal disturbances, general physical weakness, or poor chewing ability.

Note: Soft diet contains whole pieces of food that are not chopped or pureed. Some elements of this soft diet may need to be adjusted in consistency to fit the needs of the particular client (e.g., pureed meats and fruits).

Type of Food	Foods Included	Foods Excluded
Beverage	Carbonated beverages, coffee, tea, milk, milk drinks, fruit juices	None
Bread	White or fine rye bread or rolls, soda crackers, waffles, graham crackers, muffins, cornbread	Whole-grain products, any breads with nuts, seeds, or dried fruits
Cereal	Refined wheat, rice, or corn cereals	Whole-grain cereals, bran, cereals cooked with nuts and fruits, hard or firm dry cereal
Fats	Butter, cream, margarine, salad dressing, gravy, mayonnaise, sour cream	Fried foods
Fruit	Fruit juices, ripe avocado, banana, cooked or canned apples, apricots, cherries, pears, all of the above without skin or seeds, dried fruit puree	Raw fruits, skins, or seeds
Vegetables	Cooked, pureed vegetables, vegetable juices	Raw vegetables, skins
Potato or substitute	Potatoes, sweet potatoes, rice, spaghetti, grits, macaroni, noodles	
Meat, eggs, cheese	Ground or tender meat, fish or chicken, eggs, cottage cheese, cheddar or American cheese, yogurt, tofu, and smooth peanut butter	Fried meat, chicken, fish, strong cheeses
Soup	Puree from food allowed, all cream and broth soups	Whole vegetable or meat soups unless adjusted in consistency for patient
Dessert	Custard, gelatin, angel food cake, tapioca, puddings, ice cream, cake, plain cookies, hard candy	Rich desserts, nuts, raisins, coconut
Condiments	Salt, pepper, sugar, vinegar, sauces, gravy, ketchup, honey, syrup, jelly	Olives, pickles, popcorn, relishes, strong spices

Adapted from *General diets, soft diet,* Bethesda, MD, 2002, NIH Clinical Center, National Institutes of Health.

American Heart Association Guidelines for a Heart-Healthy Diet 2006

The 2006 recommendations include the following points:

▼ Consume an overall healthy diet.

▼ Maintain a healthy body weight by balancing calories consumed with calories burned.

▼ Be aware of your daily caloric requirements and increase awareness of the calorie content of various food portions.

▼ Obtain 30 minutes of physical activity each day.

▼ Eat a variety of fruits and vegetables (not fruit juices) adding deeply colored ones such as spinach, carrots, peaches, and berries.

▼ Limit carbohydrate choices to whole-grain, high-fiber foods.

▼ Have 2 servings of fish relatively high in omega-3 fatty acids twice a week. (Pregnant women and children should avoid mercury-contaminated fish.)

▼ Choose lean meats, low-fat (1%) or fat-free dairy products; limit intake of saturated fat, *trans* fat, and cholesterol.

▼ Take in few beverages and foods with added sugars, including high-fructose corn syrup.

▼ Keep sodium consumption down to 2300 mg of sodium daily; prepare foods with little or no salt. Middle-age and older adults, African Americans, and those with hypertension should limit sodium intake to 1500 mg of sodium per day.

▼ Limit alcohol to 1 drink per day for women and 2 drinks per day for men. (1 drink = 12 oz of beer, 4 oz of wine, 1.5 oz of 80-proof distilled spirits, or 1 oz of 100-proof spirits.)

▼ At all times be aware of portion size; when eating out, select vegetables and fruits and avoid foods prepared with added saturated or *trans* fat, salt, and sugar.

Adapted from AHA Dietary and Lifestyle Recommendations Revised. Available at www.medscape.com/viewarticle/536831?src=nursecenl (accessed July 20, 2006).

Guidelines for Low-Fat Diets

Frequently Consumed High-Fat Foods	Alternative Foods
Fried foods	Roast, bake, grill, stir-fry, or broil foods when possible
	Baste meats with broth or stock
	Use nonstick cookware and an aerosol cooking spray
Fatty meats (bacon, sausage, choice grade meats, frankfurters, luncheon meats)	Choose 2 or 3 servings of meat, poultry, shellfish or fish with a daily total of about 6 oz
	Choose a vegetarian entrée (dried beans and peas) at least once a week

Continued

Guidelines for Low-Fat Diets—cont'd

Frequently Consumed High-Fat Foods	Alternative Foods
	Trim visible fat from meat; remove skin from poultry before eating
	Choose beef grade "select" because it contains less fat marbling; leaner cuts of meat include flank, sirloin or tenderloin, loin pork chops
	Marinate leaner cuts of meat in lemon juice, flavored vinegars, or fruit juices
Cheese (aged cheese and cream cheese)	Choose cheese with 6 g or less of fat per ounce such as Farmer's cheese
High-fat snacks (chips, some crackers, dips)	Substitute pretzels, low-fat crackers, air-popped popcorn
Salad dressing, mayonnaise, sour cream	Use fat-free or reduced-fat salad dressings and sour cream
	Substitute plain low-fat yogurt for mayonnaise or sour cream
	Rely on mustard and salad greens to add moisture to sandwiches rather than high-fat spreads
Gravies	Use the paste method for making gravy or sauces (add flour or cornstarch to cold liquids slowly and blend well)
Homogenized whole milk products	Use skim milk, buttermilk, low-fat yogurt, and cottage cheese
Margarine and seasonings such as lard, bacon, or ham	Use jam, jelly, or marmalade spread instead of butter or margarine
	Season with herbs, lemon juice, or stock rather than lard, bacon, or ham
Breads and cereals	Plain bread, rolls, graham crackers, matzoh, saltines, pretzels, most cereals

THE DASH DIET

The DASH "combination diet" was shown by research to lower blood pressure and therefore may help prevent and control high blood pressure.

The "combination diet" is rich in fruits, vegetables, and low-fat dairy foods, and low in saturated and total fat. It also is low in cholesterol; high in dietary fiber, potassium, calcium, and magnesium; and moderately high in protein.

The DASH eating plan on the next page is based on 2000 calories a day. Depending on caloric needs, the number of daily servings in a food group may vary from those listed.

Food Group	Daily Servings	Serving Sizes	Examples and Notes	Significance of Each Food Group to the DASH Diet Pattern
Grains and grain products	7-8	1 slice bread $\frac{1}{2}$ C dry cereal $\frac{1}{2}$ C cooked rice, pasta, or cereal	Whole wheat bread, English muffin, pita bread, bagel, cereals, grits, oatmeal	Major sources of energy and fiber
Vegetables	4-5	1 C raw leafy vegetable $\frac{1}{2}$ C cooked vegetable 6 oz vegetable juice	Tomatoes, potatoes, carrots, peas, squash, broccoli, turnip greens, collards, kale, spinach, artichokes, sweet potatoes, beans	Rich sources of potassium, magnesium, and fiber
Fruits	4-5	6 oz fruit juice 1 medium fruit $\frac{1}{4}$ C dried fruit $\frac{1}{2}$ C fresh, frozen, or canned fruit	Apricots, bananas, dates, oranges, orange juice, grapefruit, grapefruit juice, mangoes, melons, peaches, pineapples, prunes, raisins, strawberries, tangerines	Important sources of potassium, magnesium, and fiber
Low-fat or nonfat dairy foods	2-3	8 oz milk 1 C yogurt 1.5 oz cheese	Skim or 1% milk, skim or low-fat buttermilk, nonfat or low-fat yogurt, part skim mozzarella cheese, nonfat juice	Major sources of calcium and protein

Continued

Food Group	Daily Servings	Serving Sizes	Examples and Notes	Significance of Each Food Group to the DASH Diet Pattern
Meats, poultry, and fish	2 or less	3 oz cooked meats, poultry, or fish	Select only lean; trim away visible fats; broil, roast, or boil, instead of frying; remove skin from poultry	Rich sources of protein and magnesium
Nuts, seeds, and legumes	4-5 per week	1.5 oz or $\frac{1}{3}$ C nuts $\frac{1}{2}$ oz or 2 Tbsp seed $\frac{1}{2}$ C cooked legumes	Almonds, filberts, mixed nuts, peanuts, walnuts, sunflower seeds, kidney beans, lentils	Rich sources of energy, magnesium, potassium, protein, and fiber

Available at www.nhlbi.nih.gov/nhlbi/nhlbi.htm (accessed July 25, 2006).

Sodium-Restricted Diet

Along with foods, the sodium content of medications and local water should be considered. Potent oral diuretics have lessened the need for severe limitation of sodium in the diet.

Indications: Chronic heart failure, hypertension, atherosclerosis, edema, cirrhosis of the liver, or chronic kidney disease

Type of Diet	Sodium per Day Allowed	Foods Excluded
No added salt	4-5 g	No salty or high-sodium processed foods; do not add salt to food at the table; use only small amounts in cooking
Mild sodium restriction	2-3 g	No added salt; no pickles, olives, bacon, ham, chips, canned soups, salted nuts, smoked meats or fish, bouillon, frozen entrées, luncheon meats, processed cheese, regular peanut butter, instant cocoa or hot cereals, cooking wine, seasoning salts, soy sauce, Worcestershire sauce, meat extracts

Sodium-Restricted Diet—cont'd

Type of Diet	Sodium per Day Allowed	Foods Excluded
Moderate sodium restriction	1 g	Same foods restricted as previous; only low-sodium products to be used; no commercial baked products, no cheese containing salt, no canned or frozen vegetables containing salt; no more than 2 cups of milk
Severe sodium restriction	500 mg	Same foods restricted as previous; only salt-free bread; no high-sodium fruits or vegetables such as celery, carrots, beets, artichokes, Swiss chard, greens, kale, spinach, white turnips, sauerkraut, hominy

High-Fiber Diet

Fiber increases fecal bulk, holds water, and binds calcium, magnesium, and other needed nutrients. The inclusion of high-fiber foods in the diet is recommended for patients on a general diet and those with constipation, and it may be helpful in the treatment of diverticular disease. High-fiber foods include whole-wheat breads and cereals, bran, oatmeal, wheat germ, millet, brown rice, cornmeal, legumes (dried beans), nuts, seeds, and fresh fruits and vegetables with skins (e.g., apples, grapes, apricots, raw cauliflower, carrots, celery, cabbage, lettuce). Bananas, prunes, dates, figs, and rhubarb are good laxatives, as well as being high in fiber.

High-Calorie, High-Protein, High-Vitamin Diet

This diet is indicated for underweight or malnourished clients. The normal diet is supplemented with foods high in protein, vitamins, and calories. Small, frequent feedings are best (six to eight per day). The caloric value can be 25% to 50% above normal (up to 3000 calories/day), and the protein increased to 90 to 100 g/day for adults who do not have renal insufficiency.

Group	Number of Servings
Milk	4 or more
Meat or meat substitutes	3 or 4
Breads and cereals	4 to 8
Fruits and vegetables	4 or more

Cheeses, sauces, cream soups, potatoes, ice cream, pudding, and milk shakes may be used liberally. Prepared nutritional supplements such as Ensure, Ensure Plus, Sustacal, Boost, or Carnation Instant Breakfast may be used at meals or between meals. Supplementary vitamins may be indicated.

Principles for Administering Tube (Enteral) Feedings

▼ Always check for proper tube placement before beginning a feeding. If feeding is continuous, check placement once per shift or before adding formula to the container.

▼ Elevate the head of the bed 30 to 45 degrees and leave it up for 30 to 60 minutes after the feeding. Keep the head of the bed elevated at all times if the feeding is continuous.

▼ Check for gastric residual before starting the next feeding, or every 4 hours. If the residual is more than half of the volume given in the last feeding, or greater than 150 mL when continuous feeding is in progress, replace the residual and delay the next feeding for 1 to 2 hours. For continuous feeding, notify the physician of the excessive residual amount.

▼ If nausea occurs, stop the feeding and notify the physician.

▼ If persistent diarrhea occurs, notify the physician.

▼ Monitor bowel movements.

▼ Check skin turgor to be certain patient is not becoming dehydrated.

▼ Be alert to signs of hyperglycemia during the first few days of tube feeding.

▼ Flush the tubing with 30 to 50 mL of water, depending on fluid requirements, after each feeding and at least once per shift.

▼ When giving medications, flush the tubing with 10 to 30 mL of water initially and with 10 mL of water after each medication. Do not mix medications together.

▼ Use elixirs rather than crushed pills whenever possible. If pills have to be crushed, ask the pharmacy to prepare them and mix with appropriate solution.

▼ If tubing is clogged, check with a nurse for unit protocol on unclogging tubing. Sometimes using warm water and milking the tubing is sufficient; carbonated Coca-Cola is used in some facilities, and cranberry juice is used in others.

6

Obtaining Information via the Internet

RESOURCES FOR NURSING STUDENTS

Care plans, care plan template, and information
http://www.rncentral.com/careplans/contents.html

Drug calculation help
http://medi-smart.com/student_drugcalc.htm

Pharmacology help
http://www.druginfo.com
http://www.healthtouch.com/level1/p_dri.htm
http://www.nlm.nih.gov/medlineplus/druginformation.html

Dictionary, encyclopedia, *Gray's Anatomy*, and other online references
http://www.bartleby.com

ECG Learning Center
http://medstat.library.med.utah.edu/kw/ecg
http://library.med.utah.edu/kw/ecg

General resources
http://www.nursingnet.org
http://www.medi-smart.com
http://nurseshift.com
http://allnurses.com
http://www.medicinenet.com/script/main/hp.asp
http://www.RNstudents.com

Internet Library
http://www.ipl.org

Working with disabilities
http://www.exceptionalnurse.com

Nursing care plan resources
http://medi-smart.com/carepl.htm

NCLEX information and study tips
http://www.nursingstudio.net/2005/10/28/nclex-study-tips
http://www.nclexinfo.com
http://www.nursezone.com/student_nurse_center/nclex_prep.asp
http://www.RNstudents.com

Physical examination—The Auscultation Assistant
http://www.wilkes.med.ucla.edu/intro.html
http://ruby.fgcu.edu/courses/80277/Intro/index.htm
http://medicine.ucsd.edu/clinicalimg/
http://health.discovery.com/tools/blausen/blausen.html
http://www.ltcpractice.com/content/node-6/clinicians/guide.htm
http://medinfo.ufl.edu/year1/bcs/clist/index.html

Cultural information
http://erc.msh.org/mainpage.cfm?file=1.0.htm&module=provider&
language=English
http://www.culturediversity.org

Cardiac sites on all aspects of the heart
http://www.fi.edu/biosci
http://heartcenteronline.com
http://www.meddean.luc.edu/lumen/meded/medicine/pulmonar/
pd/pstep39.htm
http://home.case.edu/~dck3/heart/listen.html
http://www.sci.sdsu.edu/multimedia/heartsounds

Resume and interview tips
http://www.careerbuilder.com/JobSeeker/careerbytes/CBArticle.as
px?articleID=579&lr=cbmedism
http://resume.monster.com/restips/healthcare
http://www.free-resume-tips.com/resumetips/healthcare.html

Distance learning and degree programs
http://www.phoenixdegreesonline.com (Phoenix University)
http://www.universityalliance.com (Jacksonville University and others)
http://www.college-net.com/nursing/medismartrn/- (The College
Network)
http://medi-smart.com/schools.htm (Directory of Degree Programs)
http://www.excelsior.edu

Scholarship information
http://medi-smart.com/finaid.htm
http://www.healthprofessions.ca.gov
http://www.discovernursing.com/scholarship_search.aspx
http://fastweb.monster.com/fastweb/register/start?ref=google_nur
sing-1f

Study aids
http://www.medi-smart.com/student.htm
http://kcsun3.tripod.com
http://web.nmsu.edu/~ebosman/nursing/
careplan.shtml

Study guides in various languages
http://www.studygs.net

Arterial blood gas tutorial
http://www.nurseshift.com
http://web.indstate.edu/mary/abgdemo.html

ASSOCIATIONS

Alzheimer's Association
http://www.alz.org

American Association of Diabetes Educators
http://www.aadenet.org

American Cancer Society
http://www.cancer.org/docroot/home/index.asp

American Diabetes Association
http://www.diabetes.org

American Foundation for the Blind
http://www.afb.org

American Heart Association
http://americanheart.org

American Lung Association
http://www.lungusa.org

American Nurses Association
http://www.nursingworld.org

Arthritis Foundation
http://www.arthritis.org

Deafness Research Foundation
http://www.drf.org

Endometriosis Organization
http://www.endometriosisassn.org/press3.html

Epilepsy Foundation of America
http://www.epilepsyfoundation.org

Leukemia Society of America
http://www.leukemia.org

Multiple Sclerosis Association of America
http://msaa.com

National Association for Continence
http://www.nafc.org

National Federation of Licensed Practical Nurses
http://www.nflpn.org/about.html

National Headache Association
http://www.headaches.org

**National Heart, Lung, and Blood Institute
(blood pressure information)**
http://www.nhlbi.nih.gov

National Kidney Foundation
http://www.kidney.org

National Multiple Sclerosis Society
http://www.nmss.org

National Parkinson's Foundation
http://parkinson.org

National Stroke Organization
http://www.stroke.org

National Student Nurses Association
http://www.nsna.org

Parkinson's Disease Foundation
http://www.pdf.org

Simon Foundation for Continence
http://www.simonfoundation.org

United Ostomy Association of America
http://www.uoaa.org

NUTRITION RESOURCES

American Dietetic Association
http://www.eatright.org

Arbor Nutrition Guide
http://arborcom.com

Diabetic recipes
http://www.recipesource.com/special-diets/diabetic

Dietary guidelines for the chronic obstructive pulmonary disease (COPD) patient
http://www.aarc.org/patient_education/tips/copd.html

Vitamin List
http://www.cncplan.com/vitamins.htm

CONTINUING EDUCATION

http://www.meniscus.com/web/frames/fseduprof.htm
http://www.medscape.com/nurseshome
http://www.nurse.com/ce
http://nursingworld.org/ce/cehome.cfm
http://www.nursingcenter.com/prodev/ce_online.asp
http://www.ceu4u.com/medi-smart
http://www2cecity.com
http://www.rn.com
http://www.cmezone.com

DISEASE INFORMATION AND PATIENT TEACHING MATERIALS

Allergy and Asthma Rochester Resource Center
http://www.allallergy.net/organizations/orgarticles.cfm?rytunet=
AARRC

Asthma and allergy resources
http://www.aafa.org

Cancer patient resources
http://www.cancer-info.com
http://www.cancer.gov
http://www.acor.org/types.html
http://www.oncolink.upenn.edu

Caregiver information
http://www.caregiver.comhttp://www.caregiver.org/caregiver/
jsp/home.jsp

Clinical practice guidelines
http://www.ahrq.gov/clinic/cpgsix.htm

Diabetes education and information sites
http://www.joslin.harvard.edu
http://diabetes.niddk.nih.gov
http://www.diabetesmonitor.com
http://www.diabetesinc.org/indexa.htm
http://www.diabetes-self-mgmt.com
http://www.healthcentral.com/ diabetes/?ic=1102

Disability Resource Center
http://www.blvd.com/accent

Caring Connections (end of life care)
http://www.caringinfo.org

Healthtouch (health resource directory)
http://www.healthtouch.com

Healthy World
http://www.healthy.net

Heart information risk assessment and patient teaching materials
http://www. heart.health.ivillage.com/index.cfm

HIV/AIDS treatment information service
http://www.aidsinfo.nih.gov
http://hivinsite.ucsf.edu

Infection and disease control
http://www.cdc.gov
http://www.nlm.nih.gov/medlineplus/infectioncontrol.html

IntelliHealth
http://www.intelihealth.com

Laboratory Tests
http://www.labtestsonline.org

Mayo Clinic resources
http://www.mayoclinic.com

Medical information resources
http://www.mayoclinic.org/healthinfo
http://health.nih.gov
http://www.healthcentral.com

Medline Plus
http://medlineplus.gov

Mended Hearts, Inc.
http://www.mendedhearts.org

Migraine Resource Center
http://www.migrainehelp.com

National Hospice and Palliative Care Organization
http://www. nhpco.org/templates/1/homepage.cfm

National Institute on Aging
http://www.nia.nih.gov

**National Institute of Arthritis and Musculoskeletal
and Skin Diseases**
http://www.niams.nih.gov/an/index.htm

National Institutes of Health
http://www.nih.gov

National Sleep Foundation
http://www.sleepfoundation.org

National Women's Health Information Center
http://www.4women.gov

North American Menopause Society
http://www.menopause.org

Pain resources
http://www.aapainmanage.org
http://www.theacpa.org
http://www.painandhealth.org/cancer-links.html
http://www.painfoundation.org/Parkinson's Disease
information
http://www.MyParkinsons.com

Patient education materials
http://medicalcenter.osu.edu/patientcare/healthinformation/
education/index.cfm?CFID=19402512&CFTOKEN=81963681

Patient handouts
http://familydoctor.org/770.xml
http://www.aap.org/topics.html

Patient teaching–health handouts
  http://www.ucsfhealth.org/adult/edu/index.html
  http://www.healthfinder.gov

Self-help for hard of hearing people
  http://www.shhh.org

Spine Health
  http://www.spine-health.com

Stress and Sleep Problem Resources
  http://www.mckinley.uiuc.edu/Handouts/sleep_guide.html
  http://www.texasback.com

Wound Care
  http://endoflifecare.tripod.com/imbeddedlinks/id18.html
  http://www.medicaledu.com/Default.htm#Information%20for%
    20Clinicians

PHARMACOLOGY AND DRUG INFORMATION
  http://www.medscape.com/druginfo
  http://www.nlm.nih.gov/medlineplus/druginformation.html
  http://www.healthsquare.com/drugmain.htm
  http://www.rxlist.com

RESEARCH AND JOURNAL SITES

Article archive
  http://www.FindArticles.com/p/articles/tn_health

Cumulative Index to Nursing and Allied Health
  http://www.cinahl.com

HealthWeb
  http://www.healthweb.org

Index to Medical and Nursing Journals
  http://www.medbioworld.com/med/journals/med-bio.html

Journal of the American Medical Association (JAMA)
  http://jama.ama-assn.org

Medscape
  http://www.medscape.com
  http://www.medscape.com/welcome/journals
  http://www.medscape.com/nurses/journals

National Center for Health Statistics
http://www.cdc.gov/nchs

National Library of Medicine
http://www.nlm.nih.gov

New England Journal of Medicine
http://content.nejm.org

OTHER SITES

To locate other sites, use one of the following search engines:

AltaVista	http://www.altavista.com
Ask	http://www.ask.com/index.asp
Dogpile	http://www.dogpile.com
Excite	http://www.excite.com
Google	http://www.google.com
MetaCrawler	http://www.metacrawler.com
Yahoo	http://www.yahoo.com

Please be aware that websites come and go. These are in operation at the time of this writing.

Appendix A

NURSING OUTCOMES CLASSIFICATION (NOC) OUTCOME LABELS*

Abuse Cessation
Abuse Protection
Abuse Recovery Status
Abuse Recovery: Emotional
Abuse Recovery: Financial
Abuse Recovery: Physical
Abuse Recovery: Sexual
Abusive Behavior: Self-Restraint
Acceptance: Health Status
Activity Tolerance
Adaptation to Physical Disability
Adherence Behavior
Aggression Self-Control
Allergic Response: Localized
Allergic Response: Systemic
Ambulation
Ambulation: Wheelchair
Anxiety Level
Anxiety Self-Control
Appetite
Aspiration Prevention
Asthma Self-Management
Balance
Blood Coagulation
Blood Glucose Level
Blood Loss Severity
Blood Transfusion Reaction
Body Image
Body Mechanics Performance
Body Positioning: Self-Initiated
Bone Healing
Bowel Continence
Bowel Elimination
Breastfeeding Establishment: Infant
Breastfeeding Establishment: Maternal
Breastfeeding Maintenance
Breastfeeding Weaning
Cardiac Disease Self-Management
Cardiac Pump Effectiveness
Caregiver Adaptation To Patient Institutionalization
Caregiver Emotional Health
Caregiver Home Care Readiness
Caregiver Lifestyle Disruption
Caregiver-Patient Relationship
Caregiver Performance: Direct Care
Caregiver Performance: Indirect Care
Caregiver Physical Health
Caregiver Stressors
Caregiver Well-Being
Caregiving Endurance Potential
Child Adaptation To Hospitalization
Child Development: 1 Month
Child Development: 2 Months
Child Development: 4 Months
Child Development: 6 Months
Child Development: 12 Months
Child Development: 2 Years
Child Development: 3 Years
Child Development: 4 Years
Child Development: Preschool
Child Development: Middle Childhood
Child Development: Adolescence
Circulation Status
Client Satisfaction: Access to Care Resources
Client Satisfaction: Caring
Client Satisfaction: Communication
Client Satisfaction: Continuity of Care
Client Satisfaction: Cultural Needs Fulfillment

---

*From Moorhead S, Johnson M, Maas M: *Nursing Outcomes Classification (NOC)*, ed 3, St Louis, 2004, Mosby.

Client Satisfaction: Functional
Assistance
Client Satisfaction: Physical Care
Client Satisfaction: Physical
Environment
Client Satisfaction: Protection of
Rights
Client Satisfaction: Psychological
Care
Client Satisfaction: Safety
Client Satisfaction: Symptom Control
Client Satisfaction: Teaching
Client Satisfaction: Technical Aspects
of Care
Cognition
Cognitive Orientation
Comfort Level
Comfortable Death
Communication
Communication: Expressive
Communication: Receptive
Community Competence
Community Disaster Readiness
Community Health Status
Community Health Status: Immunity
Community Risk Control: Chronic
Disease
Community Risk Control:
Communicable Disease
Community Risk Control: Lead
Exposure
Community Risk Control: Violence
Community Violence Level
Compliance Behavior
Concentration
Coordinated Movement
Coping
Decision-Making
Depression Level
Depression Self-Control
Diabetes Self-Management
Dignified Life Closure
Discharge Readiness: Independent
Living
Discharge Readiness: Supported
Living
Distorted Thought Self-Control
Electrolyte and Acid/Base Balance
Endurance
Energy Conservation
Fall Prevention Behavior
Falls Occurrence

Family Coping
Family Functioning
Family Health Status
Family Integrity
Family Normalization
Family Participation in Professional
Care
Family Physical Environment
Family Resiliency
Family Social Climate
Family Support During Treatment
Fear Level
Fear Level: Child
Fear Self-Control
Fetal Status: Antepartum
Fetal Status: Intrapartum
Fluid Balance
Fluid Overload Severity
Grief Resolution
Growth
Health Beliefs
Health Beliefs: Perceived Ability to
Perform
Health Beliefs: Perceived Control
Health Beliefs: Perceived Resources
Health Beliefs: Perceived Threat
Health Orientation
Health Promoting Behavior
Health Seeking Behavior
Hearing Compensation Behavior
Hemodialysis Access
Hope
Hydration
Hyperactivity Level
Identity
Immobility Consequences:
Physiological
Immobility Consequences:
Psycho-Cognitive
Immune Hypersensitivity Response
Immune Status
Immunization Behavior
Impulse Self-Control
Infection Severity
Infection Severity: Newborn
Information Processing
Joint Movement: Ankle
Joint Movement: Elbow
Joint Movement: Fingers
Joint Movement: Hip
Joint Movement: Knee
Joint Movement: Neck

Joint Movement: Passive
Joint Movement: Shoulder
Joint Movement: Spine
Joint Movement: Wrist
Kidney Function
Knowledge: Body Mechanics
Knowledge: Breastfeeding
Knowledge: Cardiac Disease
  Management
Knowledge: Child Physical Safety
Knowledge: Conception Prevention
Knowledge: Diabetes Management
Knowledge: Diet
Knowledge: Disease Process
Knowledge: Energy Conservation
Knowledge: Fall Prevention
Knowledge: Fertility Promotion
Knowledge: Health Behavior
Knowledge: Health Promotion
Knowledge: Health Resources
Knowledge: Illness Care
Knowledge: Infant Care
Knowledge: Infection Control
Knowledge: Labor and Delivery
Knowledge: Medication
Knowledge: Ostomy Care
Knowledge: Parenting
Knowledge: Personal Safety
Knowledge: Postpartum Maternal
  Health
Knowledge: Preconception Maternal
  Health
Knowledge: Pregnancy
Knowledge: Prescribed Activity
Knowledge: Sexual Functioning
Knowledge: Substance Use Control
Knowledge: Treatment Procedure(s)
Knowledge: Treatment Regimen
Leisure Participation
Loneliness Severity
Maternal Status: Antepartum
Maternal Status: Intrapartum
Maternal Status: Postpartum
Mechanical Ventilation Response:
  Adult
Mechanical Ventilation Weaning
  Response: Adult
Medication Response
Memory
Mobility
Mood Equilibrium
Motivation

Nausea and Vomiting Control
Nausea and Vomiting: Disruptive
  Effects
Nausea and Vomiting Severity
Neglect Cessation
Neglect Recovery
Neurological Status
Neurological Status: Autonomic
Neurological Status: Central Motor
  Control
Neurological Status: Consciousness
Neurological Status: Cranial
  Sensory/Motor Function
Neurological Status: Spinal
  Sensory/Motor Function
Newborn Adaptation
Nutritional Status
Nutritional Status: Biochemical
  Measures
Nutritional Status: Energy
Nutritional Status: Food and Fluid
  Intake
Nutritional Status: Nutrient Intake
Oral Hygiene
Ostomy Self-Care
Pain: Adverse Psychological
  Response
Pain Control
Pain: Disruptive Effects
Pain Level
Parent-Infant Attachment
Parenting: Adolescent Physical
  Safety
Parenting: Early/Middle Childhood
  Physical Safety
Parenting: Infant/Toddler Physical
  Safety
Parenting Performance
Parenting: Psychosocial Safety
Participation in Health Care
  Decisions
Personal Autonomy
Personal Health Status
Personal Safety Behavior
Personal Well-Being
Physical Aging
Physical Fitness
Physical Injury Severity
Physical Maturation: Female
Physical Maturation: Male
Play Participation
Post Procedure Recovery Status

Prenatal Health Behavior
Preterm Infant Organization
Psychomotor Energy
Psychosocial Adjustment:
    Life Change
Quality of Life
Respiratory Status: Airway Patency
Respiratory Status: Gas Exchange
Respiratory Status: Ventilation
Rest
Risk Control
Risk Control: Alcohol Use
Risk Control: Cancer
Risk Control: Cardiovascular Health
Risk Control: Drug Use
Risk Control: Hearing Impairment
Risk Control: Sexually Transmitted
    Diseases (STDs)
Risk Control: Tobacco Use
Risk Control: Unintended Pregnancy
Risk Control: Visual Impairment
Risk Detection
Role Performance
Safe Home Environment
Seizure Control
Self-Care Status
Self-Care: Activities Of Daily
    Living (ADLs)
Self-Care: Bathing
Self-Care: Dressing
Self-Care: Eating
Self-Care: Hygiene
Self-Care: Instrumental Activities
    Of Daily Living (IADLs)
Self-Care: Non-Parenteral
    Medication
Self-Care: Oral Hygiene
Self-Care: Parenteral Medication
Self-Care: Toileting
Self-Direction of Care
Self-Esteem
Self-Mutilation Restraint
Sensory Function Status
Sensory Function: Cutaneous
Sensory Function: Hearing
Sensory Function: Proprioception

Sensory Function: Taste and Smell
Sensory Function: Vision
Sexual Functioning
Sexual Identity
Skeletal Function
Sleep
Social Interaction Skills
Social Involvement
Social Support
Spiritual Health
Stress Level
Student Health Status
Substance Addiction Consequences
Suffering Severity
Suicide Self-Restraint
Swallowing Status
Swallowing Status: Esophageal
    Phase
Swallowing Status: Oral Phase
Swallowing Status: Pharyngeal Phase
Symptom Control
Symptom Severity
Symptom Severity: Perimenopause
Symptom Severity: Premenstrual
    Syndrome (PMS)
Systemic Toxin Clearance: Dialysis
Thermoregulation
Thermoregulation: Newborn
Tissue Integrity: Skin and Mucous
    Membranes
Tissue Perfusion: Abdominal Organs
Tissue Perfusion: Cardiac
Tissue Perfusion: Cerebral
Tissue Perfusion: Peripheral
Tissue Perfusion: Pulmonary
Transfer Performance
Treatment Behavior: Illness or Injury
Urinary Continence
Urinary Elimination
Vision Compensation Behavior
Vital Signs
Weight: Body Mass
Weight Control
Will to Live
Wound Healing: Primary Intention
Wound Healing: Secondary Intention

Appendix B

NURSING INTERVENTIONS CLASSIFICATION (NIC) INTERVENTION LABELS*

Abuse Protection Support
Abuse Protection Support: Child
Abuse Protection Support: Domestic
  Partner
Abuse Protection Support: Elder
Abuse Protection Support: Religious
Acid-Base Management
Acid-Base Management: Metabolic
  Acidosis
Acid-Base Management: Metabolic
  Alkalosis
Acid-Base Management: Respiratory
  Acidosis
Acid-Base Management: Respiratory
  Alkalosis
Acid-Base Monitoring
Active Listening
Activity Therapy
Acupressure
Admission Care
Airway Insertion and Stabilization
Airway Management
Airway Suctioning
Allergy Management
Amnioinfusion
Amputation Care
Analgesic Administration
Analgesic Administration:
  Intraspinal
Anaphylaxis Management
Anesthesia Administration
Anger Control Assistance
Animal-Assisted Therapy
Anticipatory Guidance
Anxiety Reduction
Area Restriction
Art Therapy

Artificial Airway Management
Aspiration Precautions
Assertiveness Training
Asthma Management
Attachment Promotion
Autogenic Training
Autotransfusion
Bathing
Bed Rest Care
Bedside Laboratory Testing
Behavior Management
Behavior Management:
  Overactivity/Inattention
Behavior Management: Self-Harm
Behavior Management: Sexual
Behavior Modification
Behavior Modification: Social Skills
Bibliotherapy
Biofeedback
Bioterrorism Preparedness
Birthing
Bladder Irrigation
Bleeding Precautions
Bleeding Reduction
Bleeding Reduction: Antepartum
  Uterus
Bleeding Reduction: Gastrointestinal
Bleeding Reduction: Nasal
Bleeding Reduction: Postpartum
  Uterus
Bleeding Reduction: Wound
Blood Products Administration
Body Image Enhancement
Body Mechanics Promotion
Bottle Feeding
Bowel Incontinence Care
Bowel Incontinence Care: Encopresis

---

*From Dochterman JM, Bulechek GM, editors: *Nursing Interventions Classification (NIC)*, ed 4, St Louis, 2004, Mosby.

Bowel Irrigation
Bowel Management
Bowel Training
Breast Examination
Breastfeeding Assistance
Calming Technique
Capillary Blood Sample
Cardiac Care
Cardiac Care: Acute
Cardiac Care: Rehabilitative
Cardiac Precautions
Caregiver Support
Case Management
Cast Care: Maintenance
Cast Care: Wet
Cerebral Edema Management
Cerebral Perfusion Promotion
Cesarean Section Care
Chemical Restraint
Chemotherapy Management
Chest Physiotherapy
Childbirth Preparation
Circulatory Care Arterial
   Insufficiency
Circulatory Care: Mechanical Assist
   Device
Circulatory Care: Venous
   Insufficiency
Circulatory Precautions
Code Management
Cognitive Restructuring
Cognitive Stimulation
Communicable Disease Management
Communication Enhancement:
   Hearing Deficit
Communication Enhancement:
   Speech Deficit
Communication Enhancement:
   Visual Deficit
Community Disaster Preparedness
Community Health Development
Complex Relationship Building
Conflict Mediation
Constipation/Impaction
   Management
Consultation
Contact Lens Care
Controlled Substance Checking
Coping Enhancement
Cost Containment
Cough Enhancement
Counseling

Crisis Intervention
Critical Path Development
Culture Brokerage
Cutaneous Stimulation
Decision-Making Support
Delegation
Delirium Management
Delusion Management
Dementia Management
Dementia Management: Bathing
Developmental Care
Developmental Enhancement:
   Adolescent
Developmental Enhancement:
   Child
Diarrhea Management
Diet Staging
Discharge Planning
Distraction
Documentation
Dressing
Dying Care
Dysreflexia Management
Dysrhythmia Management
Ear Care
Eating Disorders Management
Electroconvulsive Therapy (ECT)
   Management
Electrolyte Management
Electrolyte Management:
   Hypercalcemia
Electrolyte Management:
   Hyperkalemia
Electrolyte Management:
   Hypermagnesemia
Electrolyte Management:
   Hypernatremia
Electrolyte Management:
   Hyperphosphatemia
Electrolyte Management:
   Hypocalcemia
Electrolyte Management:
   Hypokalemia
Electrolyte Management:
   Hypomagnesemia
Electrolyte Management:
   Hyponatremia
Electrolyte Management:
   Hypophosphatemia
Electrolyte Monitoring
Electronic Fetal Monitoring:
   Antepartum

Electronic Fetal Monitoring: Intrapartum
Elopement Precautions
Embolus Care: Peripheral
Embolus Care: Pulmonary
Embolus Precautions
Emergency Care
Emergency Cart Checking
Emotional Support
Endotracheal Extubation
Energy Management
Enteral Tube Feeding
Environmental Management
Environmental Management: Attachment Process
Environmental Management: Comfort
Environmental Management: Community
Environmental Management: Home Preparation
Environmental Management: Safety
Environmental Management: Violence Prevention
Environmental Management: Worker Safety
Environmental Risk Protection
Examination Assistance
Exercise Promotion
Exercise Promotion: Strength Training
Exercise Promotion: Stretching
Exercise Therapy: Ambulation
Exercise Therapy: Balance
Exercise Therapy: Joint Mobility
Exercise Therapy: Muscle Control
Eye Care
Fall Prevention
Family Integrity Promotion
Family Integrity Promotion: Childbearing Family
Family Involvement Promotion
Family Mobilization
Family Planning: Contraception
Family Planning: Infertility
Family Planning: Unplanned Pregnancy
Family Presence Facilitation
Family Process Maintenance
Family Support
Family Therapy
Feeding
Fertility Preservation
Fever Treatment
Financial Resource Assistance
Fire-Setting Precautions
First Aid
Fiscal Resource Management
Flatulence Reduction
Fluid/Electrolyte Management
Fluid Monitoring
Fluid Resuscitation
Foot Care
Forgiveness Facilitation
Gastrointestinal Intubation
Genetic Counseling
Grief Work Facilitation
Grief Work Facilitation: Perinatal Death
Guilt Work Facilitation
Hair Care
Hallucination Management
Health Care Information Exchange
Health Education
Health Policy Monitoring
Health Screening
Health System Guidance
Heat Exposure Treatment
Heat/Cold Application
Hemodialysis Therapy
Hemodynamic Regulation
Hemofiltration Therapy
Hemorrhage Control
High-Risk Pregnancy Care
Home Maintenance Assistance
Hope Instillation
Hormone Replacement Therapy
Humor
Hyperglycemia Management
Hypervolemia Management
Hypnosis
Hypoglycemia Management
Hypothermia Treatment
Hypovolemia Management
Immunization/Vaccination Management
Impulse Control Training
Incident Reporting
Incision Site Care
Infant Care
Infection Control
Infection Control: Intraoperative
Infection Protection
Insurance Authorization

Intracranial Pressure (ICP) Monitoring
Intrapartal Care
Intrapartal Care: High-Risk Delivery
Intravenous (IV) Insertion
Intravenous (IV) Therapy
Invasive Hemodynamic Monitoring
Kangaroo Care
Labor Induction
Labor Suppression
Laboratory Data Interpretation
Lactation Counseling
Lactation Suppression
Laser Precautions
Latex Precautions
Learning Facilitation
Learning Readiness Enhancement
Leech Therapy
Limit Setting
Lower Extremity Monitoring
Malignant Hyperthermia Precautions
Mechanical Ventilation
Mechanical Ventilatory Weaning
Medication Administration
Medication Administration: Ear
Medication Administration: Enteral
Medication Administration: Eye
Medication Administration: Inhalation
Medication Administration: Interpleural
Medication Administration: Intradermal
Medication Administration: Intramuscular (IM)
Medication Administration: Intraosseous
Medication Administration: Intravenous (IV)
Medication Administration: Nasal
Medication Administration: Oral
Medication Administration: Rectal
Medication Administration: Skin
Medication Administration: Subcutaneous
Medication Administration: Vaginal
Medication Administration: Ventricular Reservoir
Medication Management
Medication Prescribing
Meditation Facilitation
Memory Training

Milieu Therapy
Mood Management
Multidisciplinary Care Conference
Music Therapy
Mutual Goal Setting
Nail Care
Nausea Management
Neurologic Monitoring
Newborn Care
Newborn Monitoring
Nonnutritive Sucking
Normalization Promotion
Nutrition Management
Nutrition Therapy
Nutritional Counseling
Nutritional Monitoring
Oral Health Maintenance
Oral Health Promotion
Oral Health Restoration
Order Transcription
Organ Procurement
Ostomy Care
Oxygen Therapy
Pain Management
Parent Education: Adolescent
Parent Education: Childrearing Family
Parent Education: Infant
Parenting Promotion
Pass Facilitation
Patient Contracting
Patient-Controlled Analgesia (PCA) Assistance
Patient Rights Protection
Peer Review
Pelvic Muscle Exercise
Perineal Care
Peripheral Sensation Management
Peripherally Inserted Central (PIC) Catheter Care
Peritoneal Dialysis Therapy
Pessary Management
Phlebotomy: Arterial Blood Sample
Phlebotomy: Blood Unit Acquisition
Phlebotomy: Venous Blood Sample
Phototherapy: Mood/Sleep Regulation
Phototherapy: Neonate
Physical Restraint
Physician Support
Pneumatic Tourniquet Precautions
Positioning

Positioning: Intraoperative
Positioning: Neurologic
Positioning: Wheelchair
Postanesthesia Care
Postmortem Care
Postpartal Care
Preceptor: Employee
Preceptor: Student
Preconception Counseling
Pregnancy Termination Care
Premenstrual Syndrome (PMS) Care
Prenatal Care
Preoperative Coordination
Preparatory Sensory Information
Presence
Pressure Management
Pressure Ulcer Care
Pressure Ulcer Prevention
Product Evaluation
Program Development
Progressive Muscle Relaxation
Prompted Voiding
Prosthesis Care
Pruritus Management
Quality Monitoring
Radiation Therapy Management
Rape-Trauma Treatment
Reality Orientation
Recreation Therapy
Rectal Prolapse Management
Referral
Religious Addiction Prevention
Religious Ritual Enhancement
Relocation Stress Reduction
Reminiscence Therapy
Reproductive Technology
  Management
Research Data Collection
Resiliency Promotion
Respiratory Monitoring
Respite Care
Resuscitation
Resuscitation: Fetus
Resuscitation: Neonate
Risk Identification
Risk Identification: Childbearing
  Family
Risk Identification: Genetic
Role Enhancement
Seclusion
Security Enhancement
Sedation Management

Seizure Management
Seizure Precautions
Self-Awareness Enhancement
Self-Care Assistance
Self-Care Assistance:
  Bathing/Hygiene
Self Care Assistance:
  Dressing/Grooming
Self-Care Assistance: Feeding
Self-Care Assistance: IADL
Self-Care Assistance: Toileting
Self-Care Assistance: Transfer
Self-Esteem Enhancement
Self-Hypnosis Facilitation
Self-Modification Assistance
Self-Responsibility Facilitation
Sexual Counseling
Shift Report
Shock Management
Shock Management: Cardiac
Shock Management: Vasogenic
Shock Management: Volume
Shock Prevention
Sibling Support
Simple Guided Imagery
Simple Massage
Simple Relaxation Therapy
Skin Care: Donor Site
Skin Care: Graft Site
Skin Care: Topical Treatments
Skin Surveillance
Sleep Enhancement
Smoking Cessation Assistance
Socialization Enhancement
Specimen Management
Spiritual Growth Facilitation
Spiritual Support
Splinting
Sports-Injury Prevention: Youth
Staff Development
Staff Supervision
Subarachnoid Hemorrhage
  Precautions
Substance Use Prevention
Substance Use Treatment
Substance Use Treatment: Alcohol
  Withdrawal
Substance Use Treatment: Drug
  Withdrawal
Substance Use Treatment: Overdose
Suicide Prevention
Supply Management

Support Group
Support System Enhancement
Surgical Assistance
Surgical Precautions
Surgical Preparation
Surveillance
Surveillance: Community
Surveillance: Late Pregnancy
Surveillance: Remote Electronic
Surveillance: Safety
Sustenance Support
Suturing
Swallowing Therapy
Teaching: Disease Process
Teaching: Group
Teaching: Individual
Teaching: Infant Nutrition
Teaching: Infant Safety
Teaching: Preoperative
Teaching: Prescribed
    Activity/Exercise
Teaching: Prescribed Diet
Teaching: Prescribed Medication
Teaching: Procedure/Treatment
Teaching: Psychomotor Skill
Teaching: Safe Sex
Teaching: Sexuality
Teaching: Toddler Nutrition
Teaching: Toddler Safety
Teaching: Toilet Training
Technology Management
Telephone Consultation
Telephone Follow-up
Temperature Regulation
Temperature Regulation:
    Intraoperative
Therapeutic Play
Therapeutic Touch
Therapy Group
Total Parenteral Nutrition (TPN)
    Administration

Touch
Traction/Immobilization Care
Transcutaneous Electrical Nerve
    Stimulation (TENS)
Transport
Trauma Therapy: Child
Triage: Disaster
Triage: Emergency Center
Triage: Telephone
Truth Telling
Tube Care
Tube Care: Chest
Tube Care: Gastrointestinal
Tube Care: Umbilical Line
Tube Care: Urinary
Tube Care: Ventriculostomy/Lumbar
    Drain
Ultrasonography: Limited Obstetric
Unilateral Neglect Management
Urinary Bladder Training
Urinary Catheterization
Urinary Catheterization: Intermittent
Urinary Elimination Management
Urinary Habit Training
Urinary Incontinence Care
Urinary Incontinence Care: Enuresis
Urinary Retention Care
Values Clarification
Vehicle Safety Promotion
Venous Access Device (VAD)
    Maintenance
Ventilation Assistance
Visitation Facilitation
Vital Signs Monitoring
Vomiting Management
Weight Gain Assistance
Weight Management
Weight Reduction Assistance
Wound Care
Wound Care: Closed Drainage
Wound Irrigation

Bibliography

Anderson DM, Keith J, Novak PD, editors: *Mosby's medical, nursing & allied health dictionary*, ed 7, St Louis, 2006, Mosby.

Anderson LN et al: Responding to difficult patients, *AJN* 99(12):26-33, 1999.

Black JM, Hawks JH, Keene AM: *Medical-surgical nursing: clinical management for positive outcomes*, ed 7, Philadelphia, 2005, Saunders.

Campbell DB, Anderson BJ: Setting behavioral limits, *AJN* 99(12):40-42, 1999.

Carroll V: Verbal abuse in the workplace, *AJN* 103(3):132, 2003.

Cohen MR: Patient-controlled analgesia: pushing for safe pain relief, *Nursing 2003* 33(11):10, 2003.

Cox S: Better time management: a matter of perspective, *Nursing 2006* 36(3):43, 2006.

deWit SC: *Essentials of medical-surgical nursing*, ed 4, Philadelphia, 1998, Saunders.

deWit SC: *Fundamental concepts and skills for nursing*, ed 2, Philadelphia, 2005, Saunders.

Fulmano J: Grace under fire, *ADVANCE Newsmagazines for LPNs*, 2006. Available at http://lpn.advanceweb.com/common/Editorial (accessed March 9, 2006).

Gold J, Thornton L: Simple strategies for managing stress, *RN* 64(12):65-68, 2001.

Grandinette DA: Help patients surf the net safely, *RN* 63(8):51-54, 2000.

Habel M: Staying cool under fire, *Nurseweek* 17(19):22-23, 2004.

Hammond S, Kelinske S, Tipton P: Going the distance, *Nurseweek* 15(4):6-7, 2002.

Hart TL: *Speedy Spanish for medical personnel*, Santa Barbara, CA, 1988, Baja Books.

Hart TL: *Speedy Spanish for nursing personnel*, Santa Barbara, CA, 1990, Baja Books.

Hawkins J, Hedrick C, Lonsway RA, Perdue M, editors: *Infusion therapy in clinical practice*, ed 2, Philadelphia, 2001, Saunders.

Hill SS, Howlett HS: *Success in practical/vocational nursing: from student to leader*, ed 5, Philadelphia, 2005, Saunders.

Ignatavicius DD, Workman ML: *Medical-surgical nursing: critical thinking for collaborative care*, ed 5, St Louis, 2006, Saunders.

Institute for Safe Medication Practice: *ISMP list of error-prone abbreviations, symbols, and dose designations*, 2003. Available at www.ismp.org/PDF/ErrorProne.pdf (accessed April 11, 2007).

Joyce EV, Villanueva ME: *Say it in Spanish: a guide for health care professionals*, ed 3, Philadelphia, 2004, Saunders.

Kee J, Hayes E, McCuistion L: *Pharmacology: a nursing process approach*, ed 5, Philadelphia, 2006, Saunders.

Keefe S: Virtual attendance, *ADVANCE for Nurses* 3(14):27-29, 2006.

Leighty J: Fast track to success, *Nurseweek* 16(5):33-35, 2003.

Leighty J: Nursing by degrees: from AND to BSN, *Nurseweek* 19(10):18, 2006.

Lewis SL, Collier IC, Heitkemper MM, Dirksen SR: *Medical-surgical nursing: assessment & management of clinical problems*, ed 7, St Louis, 2007, Mosby.

Long CO: Keeping up with drug use and safety, *Home Healthcare Nurse* 22(8): 530-531, 2004.

Lyon BL: Positive situational focusing: Pollyanna or a powerful stress prevention strategy?, *Reflect Nurs Leadersh* 27(2):38-39, 45, 2001.

Mahan LK, Escott-Stump S: *Krause's food, nutrition, & diet therapy*, ed 11, St Louis, 2005, Mosby.

McCaffery M, Beebe A, Latham J: *Pain: clinical manual*, ed 2, St Louis, 1999, Mosby.

Moureau NL: Tips for successful I.V. starts in older patients, *LPN 2006* 2(4):6-7, 2006.

National Council of State Boards of Nursing, Inc: *What you need to know about NCLEX*, 2004. Available at www.ncsbn.org.

North American Nursing Diagnosis Association: *Nursing diagnoses: definitions and classifications 2006-2007*, Philadelphia, 2007, Author.

Nursing Center: *Making the most of your job interview*. Available at www.nursingcenter.com/CareerCenter/articles (accessed April 26, 2006).

Nursing Service Organization: *Documentation 101*, Hatboro, PA, 2001, Author.

Nursing 2005 editors: Distance education: online options for nurses, *Nursing 2005* 35(2):10-11, 2005.

Pauk W: *How to study in college*, New York, 2000, Houghton-Mifflin.

Pearce LC: Diabetes resources on the World Wide Web, *Home Healthcare Nurse* 22(7):502-506, 2004.

Peckenpaugh NJ, Poleman CM: Nutrition essentials and diet therapy, ed 10, Philadelphia, 2007, Saunders.

Potter PA, Perry AG: Fundamentals of nursing, ed 6, St Louis, 2005, Mosby.

Potter PA, Perry AG: *Clinical nursing skills & techniques*, ed 5, St Louis, 2002, Mosby.

Rakel RE, Bope ET, editors: *Conn's current therapy*, Philadelphia, 2007, Elsevier.

Safety in a new town, *RN* 64(9):9-10, 2001.

Sherman DW: Nurses' stress & burnout, *AJN* 104(5):48-55, 2004.

Smetzer J: Take 10 giant steps to medication safety, *Nursing 2001* 31(11):49-53, 2001.

Strowig S: Insulin therapy, *RN* 64(9):38-44, 2001.

Summers S: Sexually charged: how should a nurse respond when a patient makes inappropriate comments?, *ADVANCE for Nurses* 2(10):24, 2006.

Texas Crime Watch: *Rape: ideas for self-protection*, pamphlet.

Tubesing DA: *Kicking your stress habits*, New York, 1981, Signet.

Ungvarski PJ, Flaskerud JH: *HIV/AIDS: a guide to primary care management*, ed 4, Philadelphia, 1999, WB Saunders.

Vandervoort AS: Washing away patients' stress, *ADVANCE for Nurses* 2(10):29-30, 2006.

Weiss B: Balancing act: no need to stress!, *RN* 69(5):53-54, 2006.

Yore M, Paljevic E, Miller M: Back to school? Nurses say: you bet!, *RN* 67(7): 63-64, 2004.

Zerwekh J, Claborn JC: *Nursing today: transition and trends*, ed 5, Philadelphia, 2006, Saunders.

2007

July
S	M	T	W	T	F	S
1	2	3	4	5	6	7
8	9	10	11	12	13	14
15	16	17	18	19	20	21
22	23	24	25	26	27	28
29	30	31				

August
S	M	T	W	T	F	S
			1	2	3	4
5	6	7	8	9	10	11
12	13	14	15	16	17	18
19	20	21	22	23	24	25
26	27	28	29	30	31	

September
S	M	T	W	T	F	S
30						1
2	3	4	5	6	7	8
9	10	11	12	13	14	15
16	17	18	19	20	21	22
23	24	25	26	27	28	29

October
S	M	T	W	T	F	S
	1	2	3	4	5	6
7	8	9	10	11	12	13
14	15	16	17	18	19	20
21	22	23	24	25	26	27
28	29	30	31			

November
S	M	T	W	T	F	S
				1	2	3
4	5	6	7	8	9	10
11	12	13	14	15	16	17
18	19	20	21	22	23	24
25	26	27	28	29	30	

December
S	M	T	W	T	F	S
30	31					1
2	3	4	5	6	7	8
9	10	11	12	13	14	15
16	17	18	19	20	21	22
23	24	25	26	27	28	29

2008

January
S	M	T	W	T	F	S
		1	2	3	4	5
6	7	8	9	10	11	12
13	14	15	16	17	18	19
20	21	22	23	24	25	26
27	28	29	30	31		

February
S	M	T	W	T	F	S
					1	2
3	4	5	6	7	8	9
10	11	12	13	14	15	16
17	18	19	20	21	22	23
24	25	26	27	28	29	

March
S	M	T	W	T	F	S
30	31					1
2	3	4	5	6	7	8
9	10	11	12	13	14	15
16	17	18	19	20	21	22
23	24	25	26	27	28	29

April
S	M	T	W	T	F	S
		1	2	3	4	5
6	7	8	9	10	11	12
13	14	15	16	17	18	19
20	21	22	23	24	25	26
27	28	29	30			

May
S	M	T	W	T	F	S
				1	2	3
4	5	6	7	8	9	10
11	12	13	14	15	16	17
18	19	20	21	22	23	24
25	26	27	28	29	30	31

June
S	M	T	W	T	F	S
1	2	3	4	5	6	7
8	9	10	11	12	13	14
15	16	17	18	19	20	21
22	23	24	25	26	27	28
29	30					

July
S	M	T	W	T	F	S
		1	2	3	4	5
6	7	8	9	10	11	12
13	14	15	16	17	18	19
20	21	22	23	24	25	26
27	28	29	30	31		

August
S	M	T	W	T	F	S
31					1	2
3	4	5	6	7	8	9
10	11	12	13	14	15	16
17	18	19	20	21	22	23
24	25	26	27	28	29	30

September
S	M	T	W	T	F	S
	1	2	3	4	5	6
7	8	9	10	11	12	13
14	15	16	17	18	19	20
21	22	23	24	25	26	27
28	29	30				

October
S	M	T	W	T	F	S
			1	2	3	4
5	6	7	8	9	10	11
12	13	14	15	16	17	18
19	20	21	22	23	24	25
26	27	28	29	30	31	

November
S	M	T	W	T	F	S
30						1
2	3	4	5	6	7	8
9	10	11	12	13	14	15
16	17	18	19	20	21	22
23	24	25	26	27	28	29

December
S	M	T	W	T	F	S
	1	2	3	4	5	6
7	8	9	10	11	12	13
14	15	16	17	18	19	20
21	22	23	24	25	26	27
28	29	30	31			

2009

January
S	M	T	W	T	F	S
				1	2	3
4	5	6	7	8	9	10
11	12	13	14	15	16	17
18	19	20	21	22	23	24
25	26	27	28	29	30	31

February
S	M	T	W	T	F	S
1	2	3	4	5	6	7
8	9	10	11	12	13	14
15	16	17	18	19	20	21
22	23	24	25	26	27	28

March
S	M	T	W	T	F	S
1	2	3	4	5	6	7
8	9	10	11	12	13	14
15	16	17	18	19	20	21
22	23	24	25	26	27	28
29	30	31				

April
S	M	T	W	T	F	S
			1	2	3	4
5	6	7	8	9	10	11
12	13	14	15	16	17	18
19	20	21	22	23	24	25
26	27	28	29	30		

May
S	M	T	W	T	F	S
31					1	2
3	4	5	6	7	8	9
10	11	12	13	14	15	16
17	18	19	20	21	22	23
24	25	26	27	28	29	30

June
S	M	T	W	T	F	S
	1	2	3	4	5	6
7	8	9	10	11	12	13
14	15	16	17	18	19	20
21	22	23	24	25	26	27
28	29	30				

July
S	M	T	W	T	F	S
			1	2	3	4
5	6	7	8	9	10	11
12	13	14	15	16	17	18
19	20	21	22	23	24	25
26	27	28	29	30	31	

August
S	M	T	W	T	F	S
30	31					1
2	3	4	5	6	7	8
9	10	11	12	13	14	15
16	17	18	19	20	21	22
23	24	25	26	27	28	29

September
S	M	T	W	T	F	S
		1	2	3	4	5
6	7	8	9	10	11	12
13	14	15	16	17	18	19
20	21	22	23	24	25	26
27	28	29	30			

October
S	M	T	W	T	F	S
				1	2	3
4	5	6	7	8	9	10
11	12	13	14	15	16	17
18	19	20	21	22	23	24
25	26	27	28	29	30	31

November
S	M	T	W	T	F	S
1	2	3	4	5	6	7
8	9	10	11	12	13	14
15	16	17	18	19	20	21
22	23	24	25	26	27	28
29	30					

December
S	M	T	W	T	F	S
		1	2	3	4	5
6	7	8	9	10	11	12
13	14	15	16	17	18	19
20	21	22	23	24	25	26
27	28	29	30	31		

2010

January
S	M	T	W	T	F	S
31					1	2
3	4	5	6	7	8	9
10	11	12	13	14	15	16
17	18	19	20	21	22	23
24	25	26	27	28	29	30

February
S	M	T	W	T	F	S
	1	2	3	4	5	6
7	8	9	10	11	12	13
14	15	16	17	18	19	20
21	22	23	24	25	26	27
28						

March
S	M	T	W	T	F	S
	1	2	3	4	5	6
7	8	9	10	11	12	13
14	15	16	17	18	19	20
21	22	23	24	25	26	27
28	29	30	31			

April
S	M	T	W	T	F	S
				1	2	3
4	5	6	7	8	9	10
11	12	13	14	15	16	17
18	19	20	21	22	23	24
25	26	27	28	29	30	

May
S	M	T	W	T	F	S
30	31					1
2	3	4	5	6	7	8
9	10	11	12	13	14	15
16	17	18	19	20	21	22
23	24	25	26	27	28	29

June
S	M	T	W	T	F	S
		1	2	3	4	5
6	7	8	9	10	11	12
13	14	15	16	17	18	19
20	21	22	23	24	25	26
27	28	29	30			

July
S	M	T	W	T	F	S
				1	2	3
4	5	6	7	8	9	10
11	12	13	14	15	16	17
18	19	20	21	22	23	24
25	26	27	28	29	30	31

August
S	M	T	W	T	F	S
1	2	3	4	5	6	7
8	9	10	11	12	13	14
15	16	17	18	19	20	21
22	23	24	25	26	27	28
29	30	31				

September
S	M	T	W	T	F	S
			1	2	3	4
5	6	7	8	9	10	11
12	13	14	15	16	17	18
19	20	21	22	23	24	25
26	27	28	29	30		

October
S	M	T	W	T	F	S
31					1	2
3	4	5	6	7	8	9
10	11	12	13	14	15	16
17	18	19	20	21	22	23
24	25	26	27	28	29	30

November
S	M	T	W	T	F	S
	1	2	3	4	5	6
7	8	9	10	11	12	13
14	15	16	17	18	19	20
21	22	23	24	25	26	27
28	29	30				

December
S	M	T	W	T	F	S
		1	2	3	4	
5	6	7	8	9	10	11
12	13	14	15	16	17	18
19	20	21	22	23	24	25
26	27	28	29	30	31	

JULY

AUGUST

SEPTEMBER

OCTOBER

NOVEMBER

DECEMBER

JANUARY

FEBRUARY

MARCH

APRIL

MAY

JUNE

JULY

MONDAY   **TUESDAY**   **WEDNESDAY**

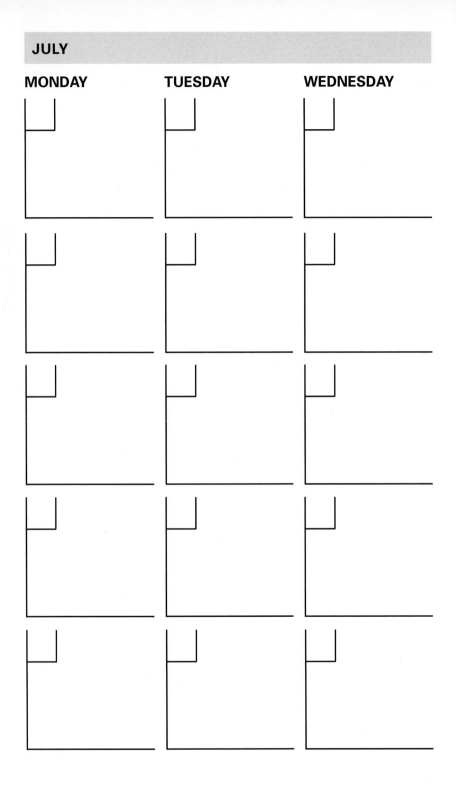

THURSDAY

FRIDAY

SATURDAY
SUNDAY

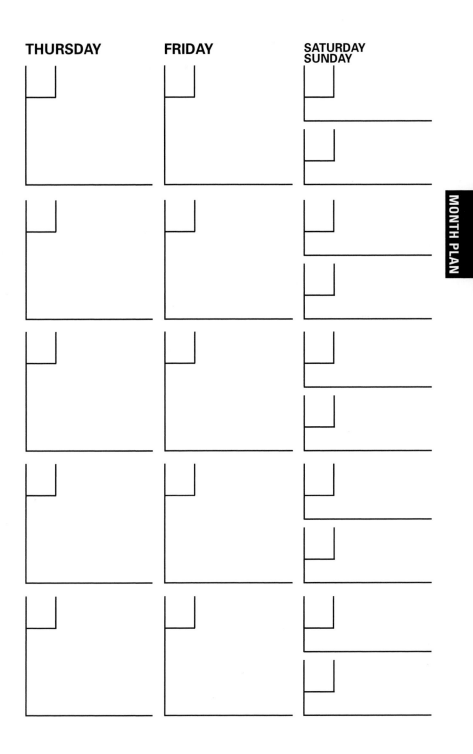

Clip for current month ✂

AUGUST

MONDAY	TUESDAY	WEDNESDAY

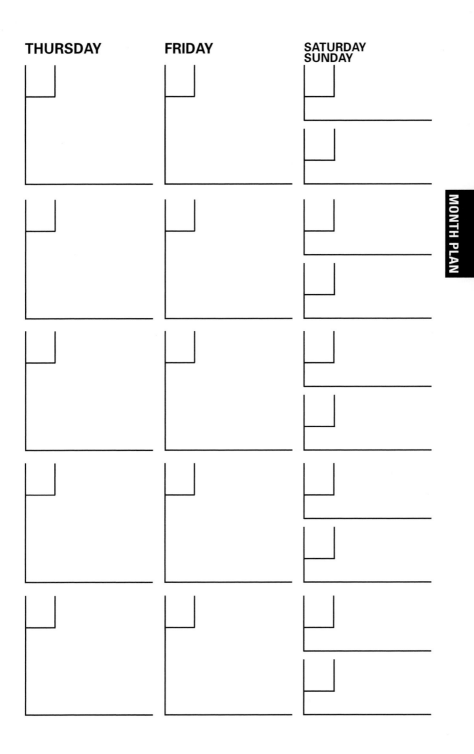

THURSDAY

FRIDAY

SATURDAY
SUNDAY

MONTH PLAN

SEPTEMBER

MONDAY   **TUESDAY**   **WEDNESDAY**

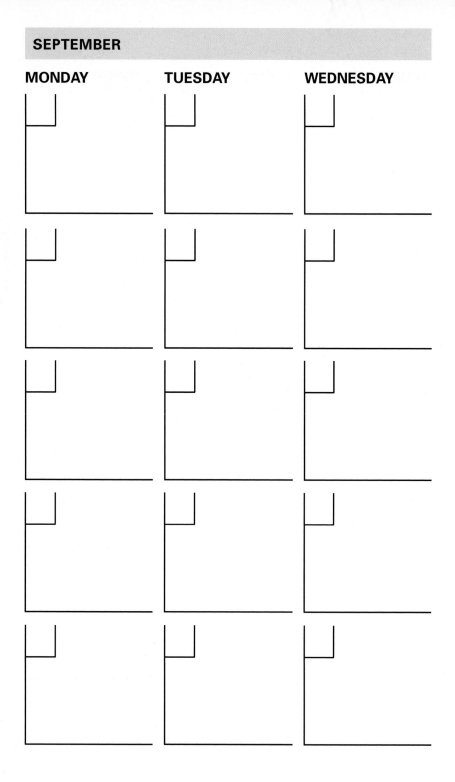

THURSDAY

FRIDAY

SATURDAY
SUNDAY

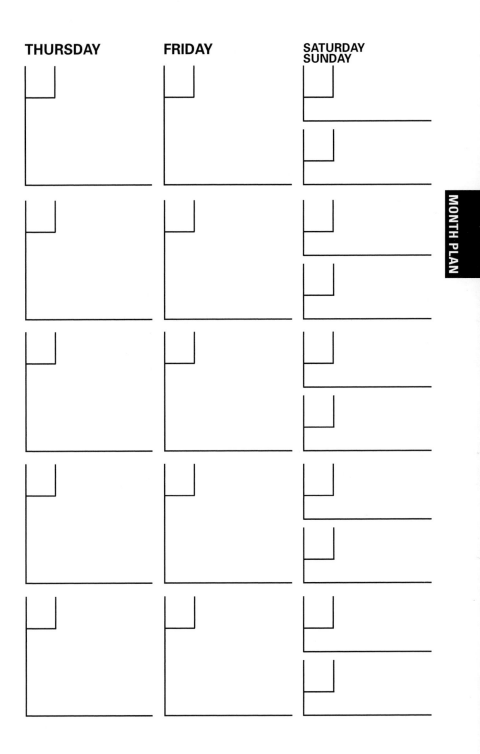

Clip for current month ✂

OCTOBER

MONDAY	TUESDAY	WEDNESDAY

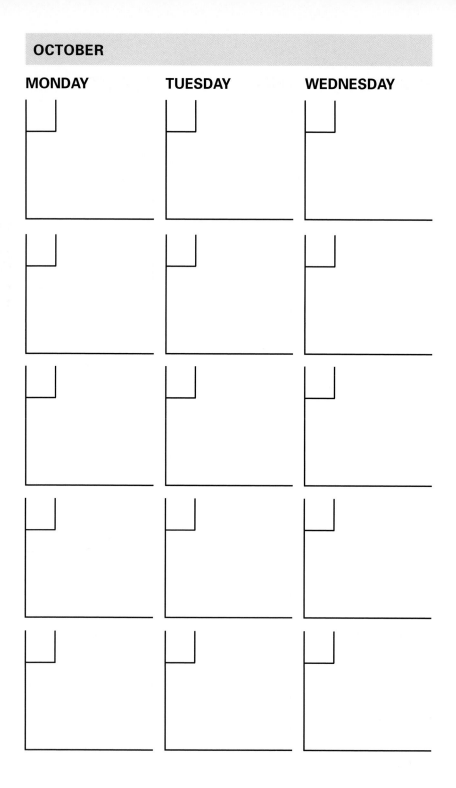

THURSDAY

FRIDAY

SATURDAY
SUNDAY

Clip for current month ✂

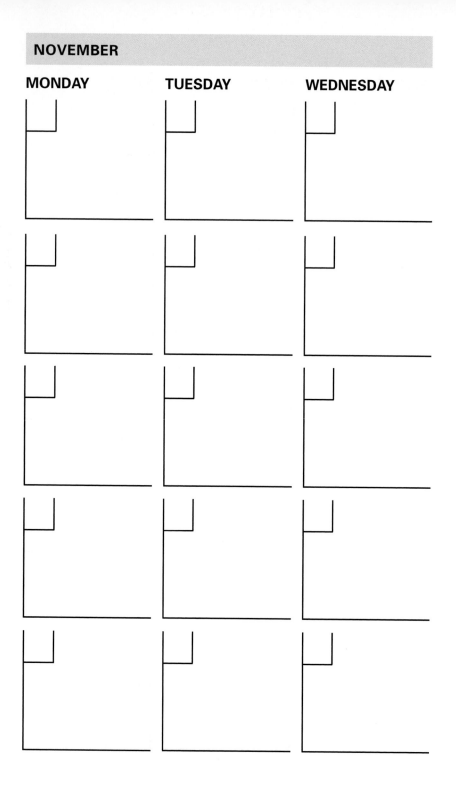

NOVEMBER

MONDAY **TUESDAY** **WEDNESDAY**

THURSDAY

FRIDAY

SATURDAY
SUNDAY

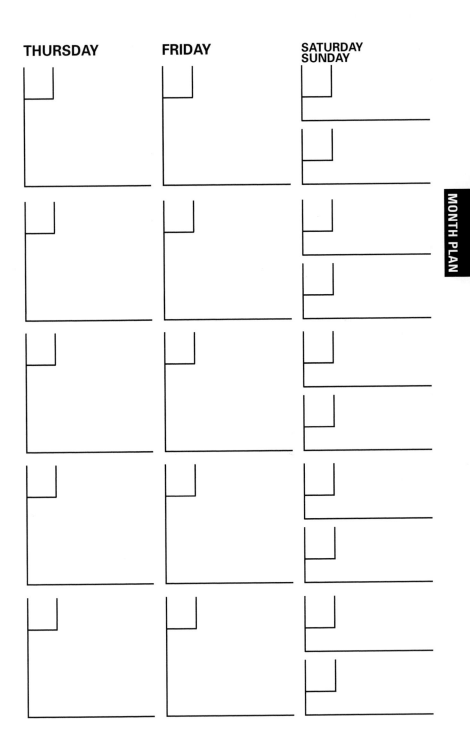

Clip for current month ✂

DECEMBER

MONDAY	TUESDAY	WEDNESDAY

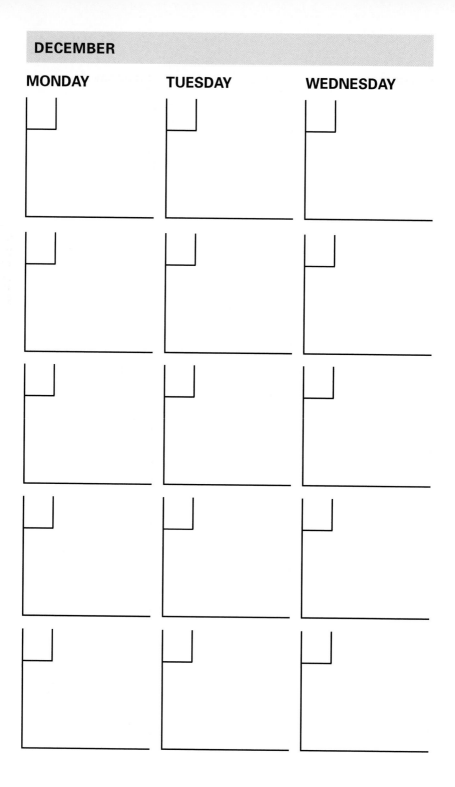

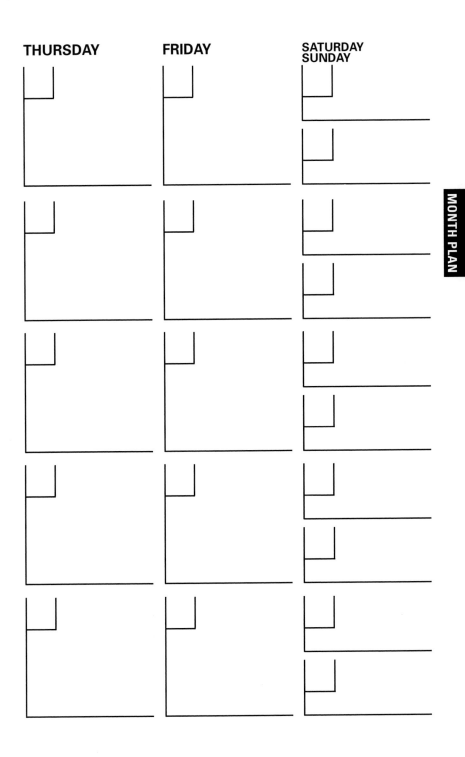

THURSDAY

FRIDAY

SATURDAY
SUNDAY

Clip for current month ✂

JANUARY

MONDAY   **TUESDAY**   **WEDNESDAY**

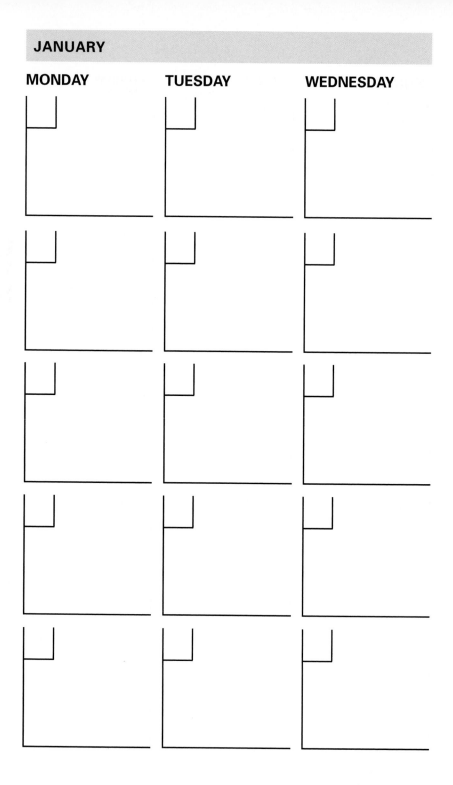

THURSDAY

FRIDAY

SATURDAY
SUNDAY

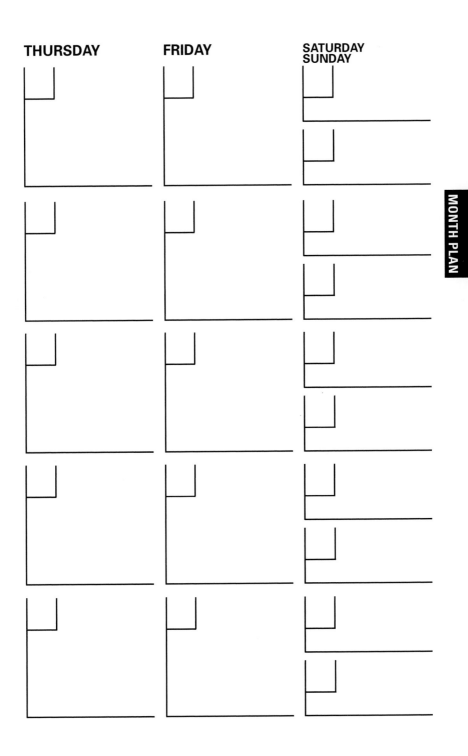

Clip for current month ✄

FEBRUARY

MONDAY	TUESDAY	WEDNESDAY

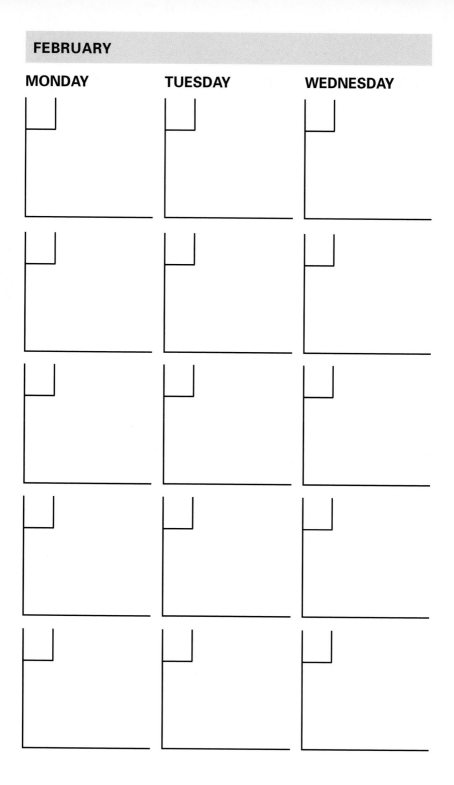

THURSDAY

FRIDAY

SATURDAY
SUNDAY

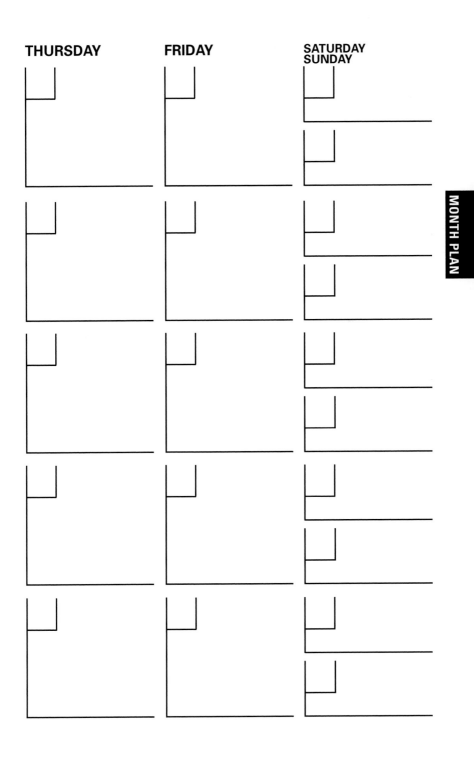

MARCH

MONDAY **TUESDAY** **WEDNESDAY**

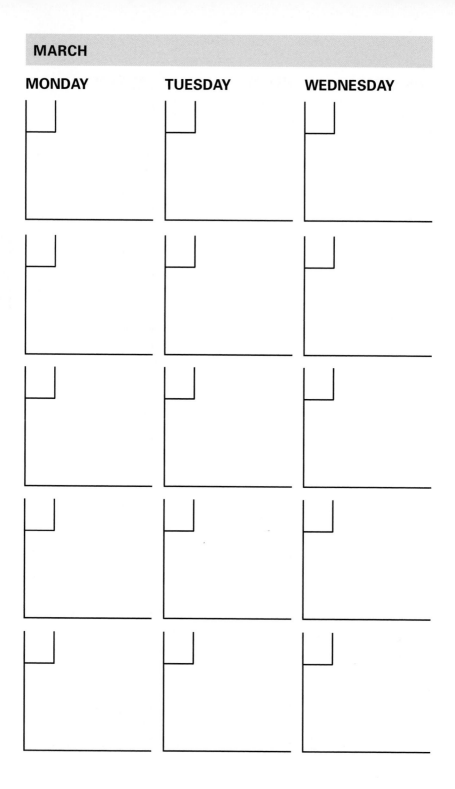

THURSDAY

FRIDAY

SATURDAY
SUNDAY

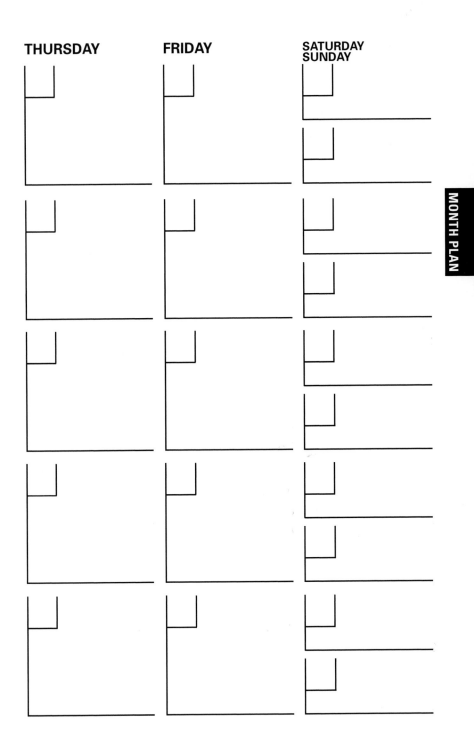

Clip for current month ✂

APRIL

MONDAY	TUESDAY	WEDNESDAY

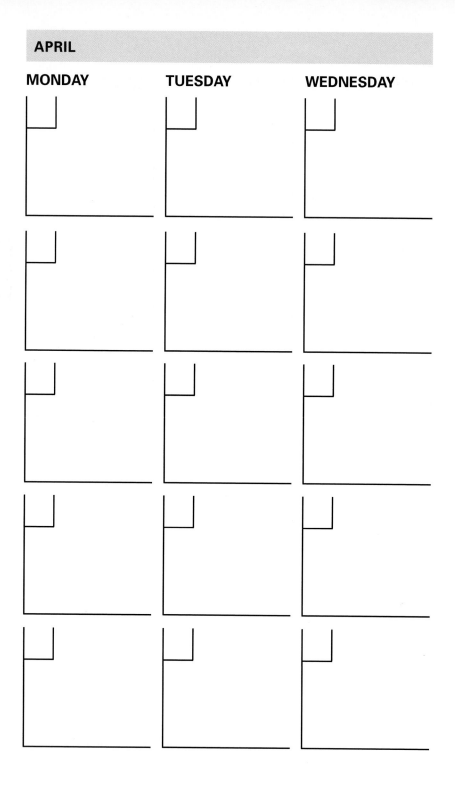

THURSDAY

FRIDAY

SATURDAY
SUNDAY

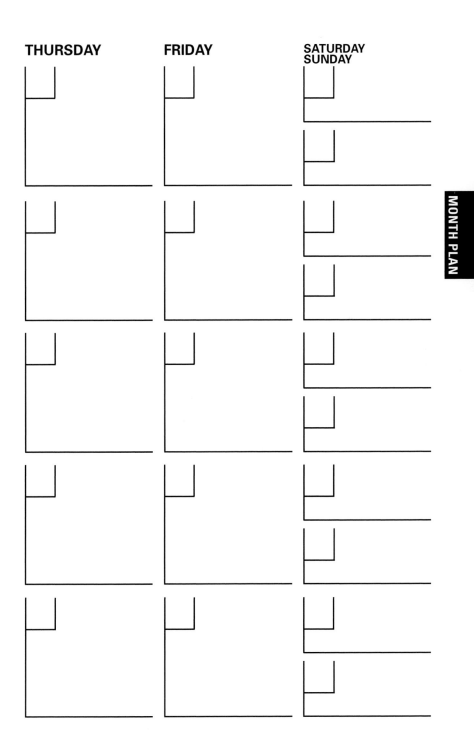

Clip for current month ✂

MAY

MONDAY   **TUESDAY**   **WEDNESDAY**

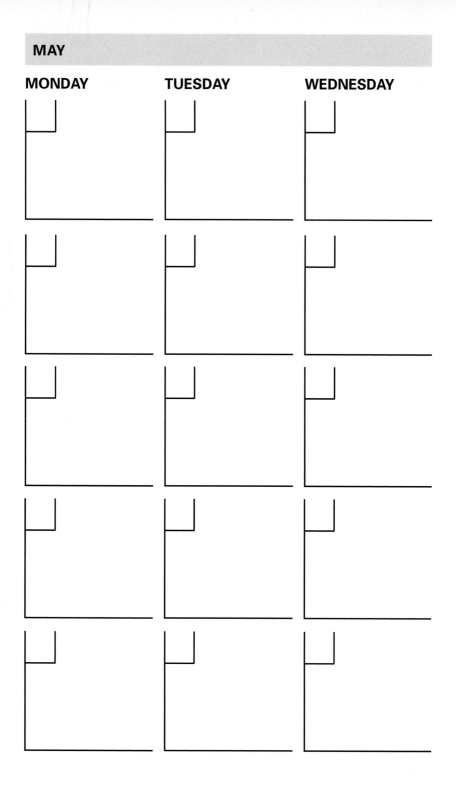

THURSDAY

FRIDAY

SATURDAY
SUNDAY

Clip for current month ✂

MONTH PLAN

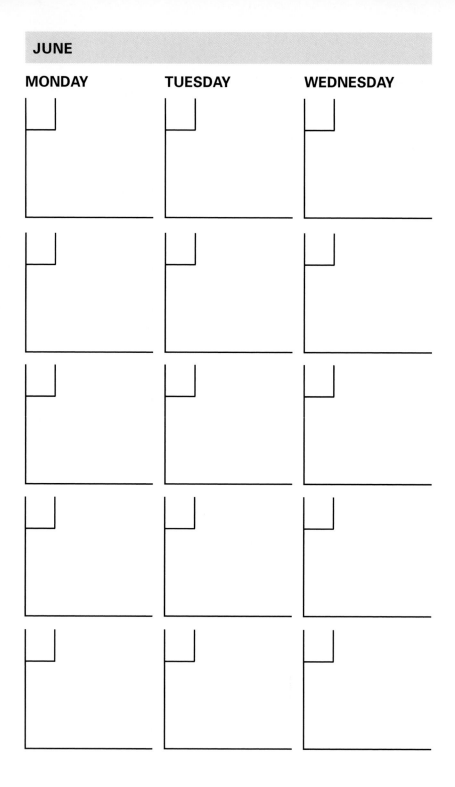

JUNE

MONDAY	TUESDAY	WEDNESDAY

THURSDAY

FRIDAY

SATURDAY
SUNDAY

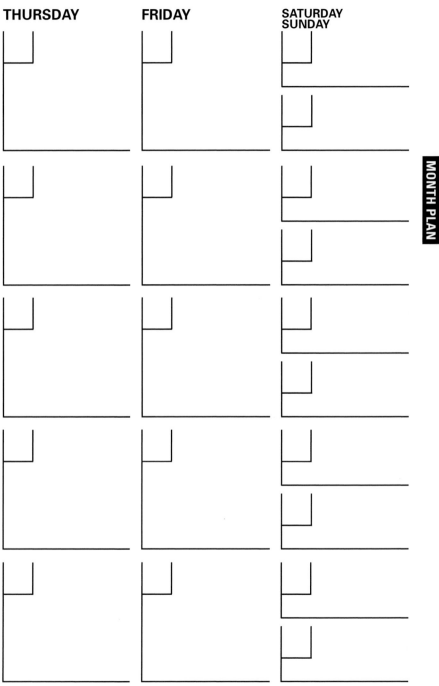

Clip for current month ✂

WEEK OF _____

	MONDAY

....
....
....
....
....
....
....

	TUESDAY

....
....
....
....
....
....
....

	WEDNESDAY

....
....
....
....
....
....
....

✂ Clip for current week

THURSDAY

FRIDAY

SATURDAY

SUNDAY

Clip for current week ✂

WEEK OF _____

MONDAY

TUESDAY

WEDNESDAY

THURSDAY

FRIDAY

SATURDAY

SUNDAY

Clip for current week ✂

WEEK OF _____

MONDAY

TUESDAY

WEDNESDAY

✂ Clip for current week

THURSDAY

FRIDAY

SATURDAY

SUNDAY

Clip for current week ✂

WEEK OF _____

MONDAY

TUESDAY

WEDNESDAY

✂ Clip for current week

THURSDAY

FRIDAY

SATURDAY

SUNDAY

Clip for current week ✂

WEEK OF _____

MONDAY

TUESDAY

WEDNESDAY

✄ Clip for current week

THURSDAY

FRIDAY

SATURDAY

SUNDAY

Clip for current week ✂

WEEK OF _____

	MONDAY

	TUESDAY

	WEDNESDAY

THURSDAY

FRIDAY

DAY PLAN

SATURDAY

SUNDAY

WEEK OF _____

	MONDAY

	TUESDAY

	WEDNESDAY

THURSDAY

....
....
....
....
....
....
....

FRIDAY

....
....
....
....
....
....
....

SATURDAY

....
....
....
....

SUNDAY

....
....
....
....

Clip for current week ✂

WEEK OF _____

MONDAY

TUESDAY

WEDNESDAY

THURSDAY

FRIDAY

SATURDAY

SUNDAY

Clip for current week ✂

WEEK OF _____

	MONDAY

	TUESDAY

	WEDNESDAY

THURSDAY

FRIDAY

SATURDAY

SUNDAY

Clip for current week ✂

WEEK OF _____

MONDAY

TUESDAY

WEDNESDAY

THURSDAY

FRIDAY

SATURDAY

SUNDAY

Clip for current week ✂

WEEK OF _____

MONDAY

TUESDAY

WEDNESDAY

THURSDAY

FRIDAY

SATURDAY

SUNDAY

WEEK OF _____

MONDAY

TUESDAY

WEDNESDAY

THURSDAY

FRIDAY

SATURDAY

SUNDAY

Clip for current week ✂

WEEK OF _____

	MONDAY

	TUESDAY

	WEDNESDAY

✂ **Clip for current week**

THURSDAY

FRIDAY

SATURDAY

SUNDAY

WEEK OF _____

MONDAY

TUESDAY

WEDNESDAY

THURSDAY

FRIDAY

SATURDAY

SUNDAY

Clip for current week ✂

WEEK OF _____

MONDAY

TUESDAY

WEDNESDAY

✂ Clip for current week

THURSDAY

FRIDAY

SATURDAY

SUNDAY

Clip for current week ✂

WEEK OF _____

MONDAY

TUESDAY

WEDNESDAY

✂ Clip for current week

THURSDAY

FRIDAY

SATURDAY

SUNDAY

WEEK OF _____

MONDAY

TUESDAY

WEDNESDAY

THURSDAY

FRIDAY

SATURDAY

SUNDAY

Clip for current week ✂

WEEK OF _____

MONDAY

TUESDAY

WEDNESDAY

✂ **Clip for current week**

THURSDAY

FRIDAY

SATURDAY

SUNDAY

WEEK OF _____

MONDAY

TUESDAY

WEDNESDAY

✂ Clip for current week

THURSDAY

FRIDAY

SATURDAY

SUNDAY

Clip for current week ✂

WEEK OF _____

MONDAY

TUESDAY

WEDNESDAY

✂ Clip for current week

THURSDAY

FRIDAY

SATURDAY

SUNDAY

WEEK OF _____

MONDAY

TUESDAY

WEDNESDAY

THURSDAY

FRIDAY

SATURDAY

SUNDAY

WEEK OF _____

MONDAY

TUESDAY

WEDNESDAY

✂ Clip for current week

THURSDAY

FRIDAY

SATURDAY

SUNDAY

Clip for current week ✂

WEEK OF _____

	MONDAY

....
....
....
....
....
....
....

	TUESDAY

....
....
....
....
....
....
....

	WEDNESDAY

....
....
....
....
....
....
....

✂ Clip for current week

THURSDAY

FRIDAY

SATURDAY

SUNDAY

Clip for current week ✂

WEEK OF _____

MONDAY

TUESDAY

WEDNESDAY

✄ Clip for current week

THURSDAY

FRIDAY

SATURDAY

SUNDAY

Clip for current week ✂

WEEK OF _____

	MONDAY

	TUESDAY

	WEDNESDAY

✂ Clip for current week

THURSDAY

FRIDAY

SATURDAY

SUNDAY

Clip for current week ✂

WEEK OF _____

MONDAY

TUESDAY

WEDNESDAY

✂ Clip for current week

THURSDAY

FRIDAY

SATURDAY

SUNDAY

Clip for current week ✂

WEEK OF _____

	MONDAY

	TUESDAY

	WEDNESDAY

THURSDAY

FRIDAY

SATURDAY

SUNDAY

WEEK OF _____

	MONDAY

	TUESDAY

	WEDNESDAY

✂ Clip for current week

THURSDAY

FRIDAY

SATURDAY

SUNDAY

Clip for current week ✂

WEEK OF _____

MONDAY

TUESDAY

WEDNESDAY

✂ Clip for current week

THURSDAY

FRIDAY

SATURDAY

SUNDAY

Clip for current week ✂

WEEK OF _____

MONDAY

TUESDAY

WEDNESDAY

THURSDAY

FRIDAY

DAY PLAN

SATURDAY

SUNDAY

WEEK OF _____

MONDAY

TUESDAY

WEDNESDAY

THURSDAY

FRIDAY

SATURDAY

SUNDAY

Clip for current week ✂

WEEK OF _____

	MONDAY

	TUESDAY

	WEDNESDAY

THURSDAY

....
....
....
....
....
....
....

FRIDAY

....
....
....
....
....
....
....

SATURDAY

....
....
....
....

SUNDAY

....
....
....
....

Clip for current week ✂

WEEK OF _____

MONDAY

TUESDAY

WEDNESDAY

✂ **Clip for current week**

THURSDAY

FRIDAY

SATURDAY

SUNDAY

WEEK OF _____

MONDAY

TUESDAY

WEDNESDAY

✂ **Clip for current week**

THURSDAY

FRIDAY

SATURDAY

SUNDAY

Clip for current week ✂

WEEK OF _____

	MONDAY

	TUESDAY

	WEDNESDAY

✂ Clip for current week

THURSDAY

FRIDAY

SATURDAY

SUNDAY

Clip for current week ✂

WEEK OF _____

	MONDAY

	TUESDAY

	WEDNESDAY

✂ Clip for current week

THURSDAY

FRIDAY

SATURDAY

SUNDAY

Clip for current week ✂

WEEK OF _____

	MONDAY

	TUESDAY

	WEDNESDAY

✂ Clip for current week

THURSDAY

FRIDAY

SATURDAY

SUNDAY

Clip for current week ✂

WEEK OF _____

	MONDAY

	TUESDAY

	WEDNESDAY

✂ Clip for current week

THURSDAY

FRIDAY

SATURDAY

SUNDAY

Clip for current week ✂

WEEK OF _____

	MONDAY

	TUESDAY

	WEDNESDAY

THURSDAY

FRIDAY

SATURDAY

SUNDAY

WEEK OF _____

MONDAY

TUESDAY

WEDNESDAY

✂ Clip for current week

THURSDAY

FRIDAY

SATURDAY

SUNDAY

WEEK OF _____

	MONDAY

....

....

....

....

....

....

....

	TUESDAY

....

....

....

....

....

....

....

	WEDNESDAY

....

....

....

....

....

....

....

THURSDAY

FRIDAY

SATURDAY

SUNDAY

Clip for current week ✂

WEEK OF _____

	MONDAY
	....

	TUESDAY
	....

	WEDNESDAY
	....

✂ Clip for current week

THURSDAY

FRIDAY

SATURDAY

SUNDAY

WEEK OF _____

MONDAY

TUESDAY

WEDNESDAY

THURSDAY

FRIDAY

SATURDAY

SUNDAY

Clip for current week ✂

WEEK OF _____

MONDAY

TUESDAY

WEDNESDAY

✂ Clip for current week

THURSDAY

FRIDAY

SATURDAY

SUNDAY

Clip for current week ✂

WEEK OF _____

	MONDAY

	TUESDAY

	WEDNESDAY

THURSDAY

FRIDAY

SATURDAY

SUNDAY

Clip for current week ✂

WEEK OF _____

	MONDAY

	TUESDAY

	WEDNESDAY

✂ Clip for current week

THURSDAY

FRIDAY

DAY PLAN

SATURDAY

SUNDAY

Clip for current week ✂

WEEK OF _____

MONDAY

TUESDAY

WEDNESDAY

✂ Clip for current week

THURSDAY

FRIDAY

DAY PLAN

SATURDAY

SUNDAY

Clip for current week ✂

WEEK OF _____

MONDAY

TUESDAY

WEDNESDAY

✂ Clip for current week

THURSDAY

FRIDAY

DAY PLAN

SATURDAY

SUNDAY

Clip for current week ✂

WEEK OF _____

MONDAY

TUESDAY

WEDNESDAY

✂ Clip for current week

THURSDAY

FRIDAY

DAY PLAN

SATURDAY

SUNDAY

WEEK OF _____

MONDAY

TUESDAY

WEDNESDAY

✂ Clip for current week

THURSDAY

FRIDAY

SATURDAY

SUNDAY

Clip for current week ✂

WEEK OF _____

MONDAY

TUESDAY

WEDNESDAY

THURSDAY

FRIDAY

SATURDAY

SUNDAY

Clip for current week ✂

WEEK OF _____

MONDAY

TUESDAY

WEDNESDAY

THURSDAY

FRIDAY

SATURDAY

SUNDAY

EMERGENCY NUMBERS

EMERGENCY NUMBERS

EMER DIR

EMERGENCY NUMBERS

GENERAL DIRECTORY

GENERAL DIRECTORY

GENERAL DIRECTORY

G/H

GEN DIR

GENERAL DIRECTORY

GENERAL DIRECTORY

GENERAL DIRECTORY

K/L

GEN DIR

GENERAL DIRECTORY

GENERAL DIRECTORY

GENERAL DIRECTORY

O/P

GEN DIR

GENERAL DIRECTORY

GENERAL DIRECTORY

GENERAL DIRECTORY

S/T

GEN DIR

GENERAL DIRECTORY

U/V

GEN DIR

GENERAL DIRECTORY

W/X

GENERAL DIRECTORY

GENERAL DIRECTORY

GENERAL DIRECTORY

ACADEMIC STAFF

ACADEMIC STAFF

ACADEMIC STAFF

CLINICAL NUMBERS

CLINICAL NUMBERS

CLINICAL NUMBERS

CLINICAL NUMBERS

CLINICAL NUMBERS

CLINICAL NUMBERS

CLIN DIR

CLINICAL NUMBERS

Index

Page numbers followed by *t* or *f* indicate tables or figures, respectively.